The Clinical Rotation Handbook:

A Practicum Guide for Nurses

by

Marlene Audrey Reimer, RN, PhD, CNN(C)
Faculty of Nursing
University of Calgary, Canada

Barbara Thomlison, PhD
School of Social Work
Florida International University
North Miami, Florida

Cathryn Bradshaw, MSW
Private Clinical Practice
Calgary, Canada

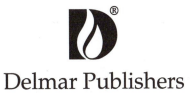

Delmar Publishers

I(T)P® **an International Thomson Publishing company**

Albany • Bonn • Boston • Cincinnati • Detroit • London • Madrid
Melbourne • Mexico City • New York • Pacific Grove • Paris • San Francisco
Singapore • Tokyo • Toronto • Washington

Cover Design: John Kenific

Delmar Staff

Publisher: William Brottmiller
Acquisitions Editor: Cathy L. Esperti
Project Editor: Patricia Gillivan
Production Coordinator: Sandy Woods
Art and Design Coordinator: Jay Purcell
Editorial Assistant: Darcy M. Scelsi

Printed in the United States of America
2 3 4 5 6 7 8 9 10 XXX 03 02 01 00

For more information, contact Delmar, 3 Columbia Circle, PO Box 15015, Albany, NY 12212-0515; or find us on the World Wide Web at http://www.delmar.com

International Division List

Japan:
Thomson Learning
Palaceside Building 5F
1-1-1 Hitotsubashi, Chiyoda-ku
Tokyo 100 0003 Japan
Tel: 813 5218 6544
Fax: 813 5218 6551

Australia/New Zealand:
Nelson/Thomson Learning
102 Dodds Street
South Melbourne, Victoria 3205
Australia
Tel: 61 39 685 4111
Fax: 61 39 685 4199

UK/Europe/Middle East:
Thomson Learning
Berkshire House
168-173 High Holborn
London
WC1V 7AA United Kingdom
Tel: 44 171 497 1422
Fax: 44 171 497 1426

Latin America:
Thomson Learning
Seneca, 53
Colonia Polanco
11560 Mexico D.F. Mexico
Tel: 525-281-2906
Fax: 525-281-2656

Canada:
Nelson/Thomson Learning
1120 Birchmount Road
Scarborough, Ontario
Canada M1K 5G4
Tel: 416-752-9100
Fax: 416-752-8102

Asia:
Thomson Learning
60 Albert Street, #15-01
Albert Complex
Singapore 189969
Tel: 65 336 6411
Fax: 65 336 7411

Spain:
Thomson Learning
Calle Magallanes, 25
28015-MADRID
ESPANA
Tel: 34 91 446 33 50
Fax: 34 91 445 62 18

ISBN: 0-7668-0540-9

Contents

Learning Tools

Foreword

The nature of clinical practice in developing expertise among professional nurses is a central issue for the profession. As clinical "guides," each of us can learn immeasurably from our colleagues about ways to improve our practice. The authors of *The Clinical Rotation Handbook* have brought together a significant set of understandings that can assist students in shaping their own learning and enhance approaches for those providing clinical learning. They have imbued their work with opportunities for learning from practice in ways that can have a lifelong impact; that is, learning how to learn is a central focus of this handbook.

Those of us who have been involved in clinical practice remember the challenges we faced, often with limited guidance and coaching. A handbook such as this would have been very helpful to me, and I believe others, when beginning the journey of learning about the art and science of clinical teaching and consultation. This handbook certainly provides such a tool for novices as well as experts.

Practitioners who combine knowledge and skillful practice are the bedrock of all professions. Practice settings for preparing future nurses are complex learning areas that challenge both the novice learner and novice teacher. The sharing of knowledge across professional boundaries, as evidenced by the work of these authors, contributes immeasurably to the interchange of ideas among master teachers, making their skills and knowledge understandable to student and faculty learners alike.

The authors ask for your assessment and feedback about their handbook. Given the heavy human and financial resources used in clinical practica, I urge those who use this handbook to offer their learning to the authors. That form of "user consultation" may help us move more quickly in ensuring that practica are parsimonious with respect to ways of achieving the best possible professional learning outcomes.

Joy D. Calkin, RN, PhD
President and CEO
Extendicare Inc.
Toronto, Ontario, Canada

Preface for Instructors

The translation of basic nursing principles and processes into practice skills is entrusted primarily to clinical instructors and preceptors who will find this book supplements and parallels their teaching. Due to differences in rate of progress through the learning stages as well as the particular format of clinical practica offered in nursing programs, this book's active learning toolbox has not been organized to fit a particular time frame. Rather, the toolbox reflects the logistics common to education of nurses. Students are then able to progress at their own pace, using the various parts of the book as they become applicable to them personally. For many students, learning by doing is more effective than learning by reading. Each phase therefore includes a number of activities, which have practical utility and will serve to improve the student's understanding of clinical practice.

A LOOK AHEAD

Nursing and health care are in a time of rapid change. Students need to develop an ability to learn and flourish in a wide variety of practicum settings. Students who understand what each practicum is intended to achieve as well as the difficulties associated with the processes of doing will be in a better position to contribute to the growth of the nursing profession and health care—immediately as students, later as nurses, and possibly as preceptors. We hope that this book will heighten your understanding of practicum learning. If, at some future time, we prepare a second edition, your comments would be most appreciated. We would like to know, from the perspective of the reader, which parts are stimulating, which are useful or do not assist in learning. Learning Tool 8.3 is our tool for evaluating your learning journey in our book, so please send it to us.

In developing this book, we have drawn on our collective personal experiences and those of our students, instructors, colleagues, and clients in various settings and academic institutions. We have drawn on the successes and setbacks we experienced as teachers and learners and those of the students from whom we have learned. We think nursing students at all levels will find this book valuable whether they are about to enter their first or final nursing practicum.

Hopefully, this book will enable students to take a proactive role in designing and managing a learning experience that is individual, goal-oriented, and meets the highest standards of the profession. If this should be the case, we will feel our efforts have been fully rewarded.

Preface for Students

JOURNAL THOUGHT

Looking back, I feel it has been a time of adjustment. It has been an adjustment for me in that I have had to change my way of thinking. Over the last month, I've learned that there are many sides to things, not just the physical facts. This new way of looking at things has forced me to think in a different way.

NURSING STUDENT

The Clinical Rotation Handbook is created with a single purpose—that nursing students who do the exercises will be more reflective learners in clinical practice. Reflective learning is an integral part of the decision-making and idea exploration process. This book is about assisting nursing students to examine their thinking and doing in practice. What and how students think affects what they do. Thus, it is important for students to examine their preferred approach to learning and use it effectively in ways that benefit their learning and care of their clients. Critical thinking influences practice decisions. It is also a characteristic of experienced nurses. We believe that the exercises and suggestions in this handbook will assist you, the student, to become a more reflective learner. Knowing and understanding the core elements of critical thinking will help you achieve your goal of being both an expert nurse and a caring nurse.

GOALS AND OBJECTIVES

The goal of *The Clinical Rotation Handbook* is to assist students to challenge themselves as well as to have a satisfying practicum experience. Students and nursing professionals consider clinical rotations among the most important learning experiences in their professional preparation. At the same time, nursing students report that practical learning is very different from classroom learning. Clinical learning requires unique preparation and critical reflection to manage the challenges of day-to-day nursing demands and situations in real-life settings. Therefore, we have written this book with the student as the primary focus based on what we have learned from our practicum students. It is our intention that this book will assist and guide you successfully through the clinical experiences of your practicum.

This book strives to accomplish several objectives.

1. The book serves as an active learning guide and is specifically written to focus on promoting critical reflection in the practicum. If we can help you become a lifelong active learner, then we have succeeded in our goal.
2. We have tried to write in an easily readable style and to organize the book in a fashion that will make this book your *favorite* nursing book. After all, the practicum is one of the most memorable experiences in your learning and we hope this book will aid in ensuring that goal.
3. In writing this book, we hope to assist in making connections between classroom knowledge and the nursing processes presented in the practicum from your instructor and preceptor. The book is, therefore, a supplement to the textbooks and manuals recommended by your nursing education program.
4. The exercises are planned to involve you in a constant process of self-assessment for exploration and self-improvement for change on your journey to becoming an expert nurse.
5. It is our hope that this book will assist nursing students to learn to reason or think more effectively about nursing practice decisions and nursing practice. When dealing with complex situations, it is easy to overlook details and lose track of your ideas and thoughts. We offer practical suggestions for analyzing and organizing your practice through five different thinking and doing processes for becoming an effective nurse.
6. The use of comments and quotations from nursing students is intended to illustrate learning struggles and dilemmas of other students that you can relate to.
7. It is not necessary to read the chapters sequentially. The book is written so that each chapter can stand independently and you can approach topics when the chapter makes sense to your learning needs and preferred learning approach.
8. This book is a practical resource to supplement group and individual learning in the practicum. Therefore, it does not attempt to teach technical aspects of nursing skills or theoretical content. It is to be used within any nursing curriculum.

INDIVIDUALIZED LEARNING

We think there are numerous unique features of this book. In particular, this book individualizes learning features for you. It is a personal book because you will write in it, and it becomes your customized textbook, acting as a permanent record of your achievements in learning. It is also one of the most personal nursing books you will own. Journal writing and the exercises designed in this book make the book unique to you. As you write in your journal about your thinking and work experiences, you will learn to step back and dialogue with yourself. Perhaps most importantly, you will learn how you learn and what you need to learn. Your practice experiences form the essence of these reflective experiences. As a *learner*, you are the toolbox and your knowledge, skills, values, and critical thinking are the tools you use to put caring into action.

ORGANIZATION

There are other nursing textbooks about critical thinking that cover practice-specific situations. This book is not intended to address each specific clinical rotation or the procedures of each practicum setting. It is a guide organized around what we have learned are the key issues and phases of the practicum. We did not include every dilemma or issue. Instead we have selected the most common questions, issues, and challenges students will face in the practicum. Thus, this book is a guide for the generic aspects of each practicum.

Content

Knowledge, analysis, and skill application tools, as well as ethics and values, are the focus of your guided learning handbook. The goal of professional nursing education is to prepare you to become a caring and competent nurse with a strong professional identity. To accomplish this you need to assume responsibility for knowing yourself—knowing how your ethics and values are tools for acquiring nursing competencies. Learning about content from textbooks is only one of the tools you need. There is a saying which illustrates the need for complex and multiple tools: "If a hammer is the only tool which you have, everything seems to need banging." Learning what you need to know is one thing, learning how to use this knowledge makes you an active learner and distinguishes you from other learners. In this way, you learn from your practice and from mistakes or setbacks. Indeed, you will learn a great deal if you let yourself examine each opportunity.

This book has several messages:

- Look for the positives in situations.
- Listen and connect with. . . .
- Look at setbacks as an opportunity to grow.
- Draw on your strengths (you need to find out what they are first).
- Focus attention on the process.
- Have the courage to be vulnerable.
- Focus on your human qualities.
- Don't give up on yourself or others.
- The helping relationship is primary.
- Performance is excellence by choice, not by chance.
- Wholeness is valued.
- Learning is a process, not an event.

Tools for Learning

Each chapter has five exercises based on the focus of the chapter. Different exercises will appeal to the preferred learning approaches of individual students. Five categories of learning tools are highlighted in these active learning exercises.

1. *Values Exploration* will assist you in developing the qualities and attributes that are appropriate for a nursing professional.

2. *Knowledge Building* will assist you in drawing upon relevant concepts, theories, and personal wisdom to increase your nursing competence.

3. *Critical Thinking Development* will help you apply your critical abilities of deciding, interpreting, judging, and reflecting.

4. *Application Enhancement* exercises are aimed at helping you apply effective skills and behaviors to your own life experiences as well as specific clinical cases.

5. *Journal Writing* exercises are designed to assist you with a common learning tool for all nursing students. Journal writing is intended to help you in three ways:

   - to *integrate* content knowledge with practical aspects of nursing;
   - to actively immerse yourself in both content and *process*—after all, it is about learning to learn; and
   - to provide a practical and *supportive guide* to the successes and setbacks of learning.

LEARNING IS A PROCESS NOT AN EVENT

The active learning toolbox is designed to take the nursing student from the process of preparing for clinical placement to practicum termination, as seen through the key learning phases and issues. Part 1 examines the context of learning (Chapter 1) and ethics and dilemmas (Chapter 2) that students may face. Part 2 addresses tools for learning. Numerous suggestions are provided to appeal to a variety of learners and preferred learning styles (Chapters 3 and 4). Part 3 assists the student through understanding supervision (Chapter 5), journal writing (Chapter 6), and other ways of constructing and deconstructing information (Chapter 7). Termination and transition tools are discussed in Chapter 8.

Student exercises and journal experiences conclude each chapter. You can use the learning tools as a reference or guide to self-directed learning; to supplement tutorials or group supervision experiences; or to complement clinical nursing courses. These learning tools include such tasks as organizing the learning plan, preparing for supervision, and participating in the ongoing process of evaluation. Students' responsibility for cocreating and comanaging their learning environment is inherent throughout the book's learning tools. This promotes a proactive stance in collaboration with the faculty and preceptors, as well as an active and inquiring learning model. Self-directed, collaborative learning builds upon each student's diverse strengths, abilities, and experience. Through this active learning process, you will learn self-assessment and gain confidence in your ability to think, ask, and reflect, as well as plan, analyze, and apply your experiences to other practice situations. It is a style of learning that will aid you throughout your nursing career.

Acknowledgments

Together we want to express our gratitude to the many students and instructors in clinical practica with whom we have worked over the years. In particular we want to express our appreciation to the students and faculty at the University of Calgary and in the Calgary Conjoint Nursing Program (CCNP), which is offered jointly with Mount Royal College, for granting us permission to use selected excerpts from journals, clinical portfolios, and assignments. A recent graduate of the CCNP program, Sue Serra allowed us to adapt parts of an information package she developed for new students (Chapter 4: "How to Survive and Thrive in Clinical" and "How to Survive and Thrive in General").

The work of Patricia Benner (1984) was foundational to our thinking in developing this book. We are also indebted to the many nursing theorists and educators whose ideas have become so integrated into current literature and practice that it is almost impossible to pinpoint their origins.

As first author, I also want to express my appreciation to the coauthors. This has been truly a collaborative project. It was Barbara Thomlison with whom the idea for a handbook such as this one originated. Cathryn Bradshaw developed the majority of the learning tools at the end of each chapter and spent endless hours integrating the manuscript. Barbara and Cathryn have enriched this product immensely through their social work perspective. As we have worked together we have all gained a deeper appreciation of what we can learn and share through interdisciplinary collaboration.

We would like to thank the reviewers for their helpful suggestions: Danielle Bellveau, MS, RN, GNP, State University of New York—Binghamton; Joan Carley Oliver, EdD, RN, Mount Hood Community College; Ayda Nambayan, DSN, MSN, BSN, University of Alabama—Birmingham; Deborah Gutshall, MSN, CRNP, Harrisburg Area Community College; and Deborah Garrison, RN, PhD, Texas Women's University, College of Nursing.

Finally, we would like to thank Cathy Esperti and the Delmar Publishers team who were highly supportive and open to the possibilities of this project. Thank you.

Marlene Reimer
Barbara Thomlison
Cathryn Bradshaw

For the Adult Health and Illness Research Group
(AHIRG)—Jim, Karen, Lorraine, Kathy, and Dot—
who share a passion for clinical practice and learning.
—MR

For Ray, Breanne, and Lynn with appreciation and
abiding affection, and for Leslie and Michael, members
of the Lazy Larvae Cocoon Club, for unwavering support.
—BT

In memory of my mother, a nurse and caregiver, who
dispensed her pearls of wisdom with the cod liver oil.
—CB

With special thanks to our students who taught us how to
teach, and to our clients who taught us how to practice.

PART ONE

Preparation Tools

1

The Context of Learning

JOURNAL THOUGHT

The first practical day in the hospital proved to be as memorable as I had expected it would be . . . On that one morning, I can honestly say that I was transformed from a university student into a student nurse. All that I had learned in the previous semester was becoming applicable and real. I have been a university student for a couple of years and I have become very good at reading text books and writing papers, but now I am applying my knowledge. I found it exhilarating to be able to relate the two fields of knowing and doing. I took in so much information that I could probably write a novel on the experience. Now I realize why I will study this profession for years — there is so much to know!

NURSING STUDENT, AFTER THE FIRST CLINICAL EXPERIENCE

You probably started the journey to *becoming a nurse* some time ago but the experiences that mark the transition to *being a nurse* come through your clinical rotations. Each clinical rotation will provide a range of opportunities for learning how to do nursing and how to do it well. You will be encouraged to reflect on:

- how theory relates to practice;
- how to adapt psychomotor skills to real-life situations;
- how to modify assessments, to develop and revise care plans;
- how to intervene and evaluate care "on your feet";
- how to handle crises; and
- how to set priorities.

THE CLINICAL PRACTICUM

Nursing practica vary widely in formats, settings, and processes. You will notice that we use the words *practicum* and *rotation* interchangeably in this book. The meanings are slightly different but both words describe the types of clinical experiences that are part of any nursing program. *Practicum* literally means a context for practice. *Rotation* has often been used in nursing because students have traditionally "rotated" through different contexts for practice, usually a series of hospital units and agencies. In most programs it is not possible for all students to have the same type of practicum at the same time. For example, half of your class may rotate from a maternity practicum to a child health practicum while the other half rotate from child health to maternity. For many nursing students and instructors the shorthand expression for the experience is neither "practicum" nor "rotation" but "clinical."

During your nursing program you will probably experience a variety of clinical rotation types and contexts. The nursing faculty who manage your program will have carefully planned each clinical rotation to be appropriate to your stage of learning and the types of clients with whom you will be working (note that when we say clients in this book we mean individuals, families, or sometimes whole communities). The nursing faculty must also consider availability of clinical resources, the degree of supervision required for client safety, and how the program philosophy fits with that of different clinical agencies. Clinical rotations occur almost exclusively in functioning settings where the primary goal is client service, not student learning. Instructors and students, therefore, need a great deal of flexibility and openness to the opportunities that present. It is this quality that makes clinical learning so exciting but we admit that both instructors and students would sometimes feel more comfortable if it was a more controlled learning environment. That is why most nursing programs provide opportunities for students to practice skills (e.g., assessment, communication, psychomotor, group leadership) in the classroom or practice laboratory. Do take advantage of these opportunities. They will do wonders for reducing your anxiety and increasing your confidence and enjoyment in clinical rotations.

Practicum Formats

Formats of clinical rotations vary in terms of the roles students and supervisors are expected to take. Initially you will have minimal responsibility for client care; the person supervising you will take the major role. However, minimal responsibility for client care does not mean minimal responsibility for your own learning! As your clinical rotation progresses, you will assume increasing responsibility for client care. In later clinical rotations you will take almost total responsibility for the nursing care of a client group; the person supervising you will then be more of an observer and coach.

Observation. Sometimes your role will be to observe clients in a particular context without any intervention on your part. This type of practicum experience gives you an opportunity to watch and reflect without the pressure of dealing with the situation. Some nursing programs arrange for an early experience in which students spend part of a day observing experienced nurses in their usual roles. The following are comments from nursing students after their first observation experience.

> This experience has changed my thinking about geriatric nursing. The nurse I spent time with was so wonderful. She was really kind, patient and had a wonderful positive attitude.

There was a mound of paperwork I hadn't thought about, charts galore. After rounds, there were many phone calls to doctors and others. We saw everything the nurse did.

Some nursing programs use observation as a way for students to compare and contrast classroom learning with patterns you can observe when watching a particular age group (e.g., toddlers in a play school). Another way that observation is used is for students to watch each other doing assessments or procedures and then to critique them. The students who observe have the opportunity to see the sequence of steps and think about how it relates to the way they have been taught. The students doing the assessments or procedures get the benefit of peer feedback. The roles are then reversed.

Experienced nurses who have returned to college or university for further education also find the observation format useful. It can help you see again what you may have stopped noticing because of familiarity and busyness. An effective learning strategy for any level of student is to write out a detailed description of the setting and activity immediately after the observation. In such a description you might include:

- the color of the walls, curtains, pictures;
- smells, sounds;
- location and condition of room furnishings;
- how each person moved about the environment;
- posture and facial expressions; and
- what was said and done.

Sometimes nursing students feel impatient with the observation format. Many of us become nurses because we are active people who want to be doing, helping, and interacting. Observation may feel constraining as a way of learning, especially if that is not your preferred learning style (for more on learning styles see Chapter 5). However, if you push yourself to make the most of all kinds of opportunities you will be surprised with what you can gain. Assessment is a major part of nursing. Learning to observe carefully for details and patterns will be of immense help in developing assessment skills.

Instructor-Led.   The instructor-led practicum format is the most common type in nursing programs. Usually you will be part of a small group of students assigned to work with one instructor in an agency, hospital unit, or district. You will be expected to plan and implement some or all of the care required by the client(s) assigned to you under the supervision of your clinical rotation instructor (Chapter 5 covers learning in a supervised context in more detail). Your instructor usually will choose particular client situations that he or she believes to be appropriate to your learning needs at that time. Often you will have some input into those decisions. Sometimes your instructor will expect you to select your own client situations within the guidelines set for that clinical rotation.

In the instructor-led format you are accountable primarily to your instructor for the care provided in the client situation as well as for your learning. However, you may also be accountable to a nurse or other health care provider for reporting changes in client situation, care provided, and needs identified, and validating planned interventions. Learning when and what to report and to whom is part of learning to be a nurse. Your instructor will guide you in this process. Sometimes your instructor or another health care provider may take over managing a particular situation if it has escalated in complexity beyond your capabilities. Your learning cannot take precedence over client safety, nor do we expect you to handle more than that for which you have been prepared.

Notes

One of the major advantages of this format is that your instructor is skilled in judging how much students can handle as well as the needs of the clients. Sometimes you will feel stretched but you will have backup from your instructor. Gradually you take increasing responsibility for identifying what you can manage in a clinical situation and where you need help. Of course you have been doing this sort of thing in other parts of your life for a long time. It is like learning to drive. The first few times you encountered roads that were slippery because of rain or snow you may not have had enough experience to detect the danger of skidding. If you were fortunate there was an experienced driver who could alert you to the danger and coach you in techniques like not accelerating on a curve under slippery conditions. One of the distinguishing qualities between novice and expert nurses is the ability to sense when there is a problem even though there are no outward signs of impending danger.

Preceptored. Later in your nursing program you may have one or more preceptored clinical rotations. In this format your instructor will not be with you to directly supervise the care you provide. Instead you will work with an experienced nurse. The idea is that you gradually learn to take on that nurse's client care responsibilities and role. This type of practicum is well suited to helping you make the transition from student to staff nurse. You will learn practical tips and alternative ways of doing things. You will refine organizational and priority-setting skills and learn about safe shortcuts as you work with your preceptor. Evaluation in this format is usually shared among you, your preceptor, and your instructor.

Internship. Internship is a less common clinical rotation format in nursing. Some programs provide a time-limited opportunity for students who have otherwise completed all requirements to serve as practitioners but with planned experiences, guidance, and evaluation.

Practicum Settings

You may have come into a nursing program assuming that hospitals are where you would practice. Secretly you may have envisioned yourself as one of the nurses from *ER* or *M.A.S.H.*, as the nurse who was so kind to you when you were in the hospital, or like your mom or any of the other nurses you have known. But nursing and health care are changing. The emphasis is shifting to more community care, shorter hospital stays, and prevention.

Nursing clinical rotations may occur almost any place where people live, work, study, or play (e.g., sports medicine clinics, schools, prisons, corporate offices) as well as more traditional health-care sites such as hospitals, long-term care facilities, clinics, and community health agencies. Sometimes students are disappointed when they don't start in an acute care hospital. Similarly, you may wonder whether you are really learning about pediatric nursing when your entire practicum for that course is spent in an elementary school setting. Be honest with yourself. It is okay to question those decisions and to talk them over with your instructor if you are concerned. It may also help to realize that, not only are nurses employed in many other settings, but also that some skills may be easier to learn in one setting than another. For example, the acute care hospitals in your area may not be the best learning environment for you to first do vital signs with real patients or to learn how to help agitated, cognitively impaired, senior citizens.

Practicum Processes

The five little words below will be important traveling companions to help you reflect on each day of clinical rotation experience. Practicum learning is a process; not a body of knowledge to be mastered as in a theory course. In other words, clinical rotation processes have to do with the journey, not just the destination.

Who.   Who did I meet today? Who will I remember? Who touched me by the beauty of their life? their pain? their skill? their compassion? their knowledge?

When.   When did I realize I had changed my way of relating to people? When did I first notice one client's sadness? another client's change in skin color?

Where.   Where can frightened parents get help for their son who is talking about suicide? Where is the emergency suction equipment on this unit? Where does this man get the strength to face an incurable illness?

How.   How can I ease this woman's pain? How can I help her get to sleep? How can I set up an intravenous line more efficiently or do a catheterization without exposing the patient so much?

Why.   Why are these parents so fearful about having their baby immunized? Why does it matter whether I draw up one type of insulin before the other?

Your Practicum Is Not . . . a Nine-to-Five Job

Be prepared for some of your clinical rotations to involve working different shifts, weekends, holidays, etc. One of the unique things about health care provided in institutions is that nurses and nursing assistants are the ones who provide continuous 24-hour care. Other health-care workers in these institutions may also be working or on call over the 24-hour period but rarely do they share the continual minute-to-minute responsibility with which nursing staff is entrusted. Other practicum settings, such as walk-in clinics for street people, crisis services, and prenatal classes, also function at times appropriate to their clientele but not necessarily convenient to students.

So what are the implications for you? Sometimes your clinical rotation hours will include evenings or even nights because there are things that are best learned on those shifts (e.g., settling patients for sleep, meeting with families). Sometimes your practicum hours will include evenings or weekends because there are so many learners in the environment that different groups have to be scheduled for different times. If your clinical rotation is a preceptored format you will be working the shift schedule (i.e., in whole or in part) that your preceptor works.

Also, because you will be sharing responsibility for client care, there will be times when you cannot leave exactly on time. Client safety has to take priority. Fortunately those times will be rare. But to reduce your own stress, avoid scheduling another course or commitment right after your practicum if you can help it. Clinical rotation time also can be physically and emotionally tiring, so allowing yourself some time to relax and reflect after practicum can make the whole experience much more positive.

You will find that preparation for clinical rotation also takes time and often cannot be done until the night before. Sometimes your instructor will provide you with information on the clients with whom you will be working the next day. Sometimes you will have to go to the institution or agency the day prior to choose the clients with whom you will be working (Chapter 4 details some of the tools to help you with this process). For now, keep in mind that the night before clinical is not a good time to sign up for Spanish lessons!

Your Practicum Is Not . . . an Apprenticeship

Apprenticeship has to do with learning a trade—learning on the job by working closely over time with someone skilled in that trade. You can see that there are some similarities but there are major differences too. Apprentices learn a trade; you are becoming a professional nurse. Apprentices do not have homework; you will. Apprentices learn primarily by doing; you are learning in a variety of ways of which doing is only one. Apprentices are usually paid because they are part of the workforce; you are not (too bad, you may say, but you have the freedom and rights of a student too). Nursing leaders have worked hard to move nursing education away from an apprenticeship model to an educational model.

Your Practicum Is Not . . . an Escape from Classes

Many nursing students consider their clinical practica the highlights of their program and that is great. However, your practica are times for reflective learning and integration of content, not just a break from class or a chance to learn new skills. Class time and clinical rotation experiences work together in creating the new you, the professional nurse.

Your Practicum Is Not . . . the Only Source of Practical Learning

Nursing students today often spend less total time in clinical rotations than earlier generations of nurses did. It is not the total hours you spend, but rather what you achieve through those hours that really counts. Time spent preparing for and reflecting on your practicum hours is very much part of your practical learning. Likewise, practicing in the psychomotor-skills lab really is worthwhile even if it does not feel like the "real thing."

Other things can also be part of practical learning. Taking part in a class discussion of a case study is excellent preparation for a later case management role. Listening empathically to your friend's frustration with his parents is an opportunity to refine your communication skills. Helping on the grad committee can enhance your program planning skills. Volunteering at a center for autistic children will give you many hours of practical experience—and you will not have to pay tuition fees for the privilege.

Your Practicum Is Not . . . Common Sense

Nursing practice is sometimes described, even by expert nurses, as mostly common sense. There is an element of "sound practical judgement that is independent of specialized knowledge" (*Random House College Dictionary*, 1980, p. 271). Your intelligence, maturity, and life experiences are assets you bring to your nursing career. By all means do use this "common sense." Sometimes when students are anxiously trying to remember all the new information with which they have been bombarded they forget the value of common sense. However, nursing is much more than common sense. Expert nurses have so integrated their experience, knowledge, and skills that they may no longer recognize it as specialized. It is like watching a superb skier who makes it look so easy.

Your Practicum Is Not . . . a Laboratory

By now you have probably had several science courses that involved a laboratory component. You arrived at the specified time; the equipment and specimens were ready and waiting; the lab guide provided a logically sequenced set of instructions; the lab instructor circulated around the room to answer questions; you did what you were to do and left as soon as you were finished. Not so the nursing clinical rotation. As one nursing student who had a previous degree in biology said, "*e. coli* don't talk back." In a practicum your patient may be called for an x-ray just as you were going to change a dressing. Most of the time your instructor will be nowhere in sight when you need him or her. You will know how to get a hold of your instructor; there will be guidelines as to what you are to do and in what sequence but, overall, nursing practica occur in settings that are much less predictable and controlled than science labs.

Your Practicum Is Not . . . Optional

In most nursing programs, clinical rotation experiences are not optional. You may skip theory classes (not something we recommend) and catch up in other ways, but not so your practicum. That means more careful planning on your part, especially because nursing clinical rotations may occur at odd hours and different places. Do you have dependable transportation? How will you get home if your shift ends at midnight? How reliable are your baby-sitting arrangements? What alternatives do you have if your child is too sick for day care? Of course there will be times when you do miss a clinical rotation day because of illness, but if you miss too much time you may have to make that time up or repeat the course. Check with your instructors at the beginning of each practicum about how to notify them if you do have to miss a clinical day. Remember too that some of your clinical rotations will require heavy lifting, long hours on your feet, etc. Therefore, the timing of pregnancy or elective surgery also bears consideration. If you have a health problem that may affect your ability to adapt to certain schedules (e.g., diabetes) or practice in certain client situations (e.g., exposure to measles), discuss your concerns in advance with your instructor. Sometimes there are concerns about clinical rotation situations that could conflict with personal values (e.g., abortion, life support). Here too it is important to discuss your concerns in advance with your instructor (Chapter 2 deals with ethics and dilemmas).

Practicum Phases

Each practicum has a preparation phase, a beginning, a middle, and an end. The successful student stays on top of this cycle, knowing how to get the most out of each phase, how to correct course, and how to bring it to a positive sense of completion.

Prepracticum Preparation.   This phase extends from when you first know you will have a particular clinical rotation to its actual starting point. Thus, you may be in prepracticum preparation for more than one clinical rotation at a time. Sound confusing? Here is an example. One of the authors of this book teaches in a program that offers elective rural and international practica in the final year. To take advantage of these opportunities students may begin exploring the possibilities and making preliminary arrangements up to a year beforehand, while they are engaged in other clinical rotations.

Most often you will begin serious preparation for a practicum at the beginning of the term in which it is scheduled. Be sure to take advantage of all orientation meetings and opportunities. Ask other students who have completed this particular practicum what they liked best about it, how they suggest you prepare, etc. Find out what you can about the agency itself—its history, its clientele, its location, etc. Pay particular attention to the specific objectives set out for this practicum. Use this information to help you review in preparation for starting.

Going for It.   Use these proven tools for success:

- check out your attitude and expectations of the practicum;
- make a learning plan;
- list the questions you want to ask your instructor;
- prepare the equipment and clothing relevant to this particular clinical rotation (e.g., good stethoscope and penlight for a critical care rotation, professional-looking clothes for an occupational health rotation); and

❧ get your personal life and priorities in order (e.g., you may need to make changes in part-time work hours, baby-sitting arrangements or extracurricular activities because of the demands of this practicum).

Evaluating Progress.   Long before now you have become accustomed to being graded on papers and presentations. Unlike exams based on recall and comprehension of class materials, papers and presentations call forth something of yourself—your ideas, your ways of expressing yourself. Even more so, knowing that what you do in your clinical rotation is being evaluated can make you feel a bit vulnerable. How do you know that the instructor is not evaluating you on personality? Is there some sort of ideal nurse role that you are supposed to emulate? How can the instructor evaluate what you do if most of the time he or she is not right there with you?

We would not be honest if we did not admit that clinical evaluation is a frequent topic of discussion among nurse educators because of its challenges. But challenges fertilize creativity. There are fair and diverse ways to evaluate students in clinical rotations. One of the core principles is that you, the student, must be very involved in that process. You will learn to evaluate yourself realistically, to accumulate evidence through journals, portfolios, and such to demonstrate your progress, and to participate actively in evaluation interviews.

Correcting Course.   By now you may have heard of the terms *formative* and *summative* evaluation. Formative evaluation has to do with the ongoing process—getting feedback, correcting course, getting more feedback, and so on. Summative evaluation has to do with the endpoint of a practicum—the final written comments and grade. Ask for and take advantage of early feedback in your clinical rotation so you can correct your course. Learning how to ask for specific feedback is an important skill for your professional growth. Instead of "how did I do today?" try questions like "how might I have handled that situation better?" or "what was I missing in my assessment?" Busy instructors and preceptors sometimes don't give you as much feedback as you might want, especially if you are doing reasonably well. Part of being on top of your own learning is asking for feedback and using that feedback toward continuous improvement.

Ending.   Ending your clinical rotation may trigger a lot of emotions. You may be relieved to not have to get up at 5:00 A.M. for a few weeks, but really miss some of the clients you worked with and the camaraderie you developed with the others in your practicum group. Ending one practicum is really the beginning of the next one. You are the continuity, the person who knows best what you have learned and what you will want to emphasize in the next practicum.

❧ THE COMPLEX AND CHANGING PROFESSION OF NURSING

You will spend a lot of time reflecting on changes in nursing and health care throughout your program so we will only make three crucial points here that are directly related to how you think about clinical practice.

Human Health

Nursing has to do exclusively with human health. That point seems obvious enough but it has a lot of implications. Your practicum is in a human laboratory. Humans are conscious beings who think, feel, value, remember the past, plan for the future, and make choices. They care and want to be cared for with the respect and dignity due them as human beings, regardless of their current state. Never for a moment can that be forgotten—whether they are a physically aggressive nursing home resident, an abusive male in the emergency department whose drunk driving just killed a young mother of four, a severely deformed premature infant, or a brain-dead patient whose organs are about to be transplanted.

Interdependence

Nursing is never undertaken independently or dependently. Nurses collaborate with clients, families, communities, agencies, and other health providers in various and often complex ways. Each of those participants bring their own expertise, resources, and needs. For example, clients are the experts in the experience, and often the management, of their own illness. As a nursing student, you may start your clinical day having some basic hypotheses and strategies about client needs and how to approach them but ultimately what you do will be undertaken in negotiation with your clients and others. Even unconscious patients give you feedback (e.g., changes in vital signs, responsiveness to painful stimuli) that you then consider in revising your plan of care. Likewise, during your clinical day other health-care providers, such as a physician or dietician, may order changes in the client's diagnostic or therapeutic regime. You may have to carry out those changes but you do so in an informed and responsible manner. That health-care provider is "dependent" on you as a direct care provider who has the knowledge, skills, and ongoing contact with the client to do what you believe needs to be done. You are "dependent" on that health-care provider whose specialized knowledge overlaps but is not the same as yours. Thus, there is an "interdependent" relationship. As soon as you step into this dynamic environment you are part of the interdependent network, even though all you may be doing is taking one patient's vital signs. The nurse responsible for that patient needs to know those results in a timely manner and those results need to be recorded on the appropriate forms.

Specialization

Knowledge and technology are developing at such an incredible rate that nurses are increasingly becoming highly specialized. However, there has been a long-standing expectation that "a nurse is a nurse is a nurse"; in other words, that nurses should be able to function equally well in any environment. In your basic nursing program you are preparing as a generalist; even so, by the time you graduate, there will be some clinical contexts in which you feel reasonably proficient and other contexts in which you have had minimal or no experience. No program could be long enough for you to do it all. But this is often a niggling cause of concern for students (and instructors): "What if I graduate and I have never worked on an orthopedic unit?" "only seen two deliveries?" "never inserted a nasogastric tube?"

So what can you do about this concern? Go for all the experiences you can get. Don't hold back hoping for another opportunity when you may feel more prepared. Ask for experiences that you have not had. Seek out part-time work or volunteer experiences that may strengthen your skills in areas of concern. For example, working in a nursing home can give you excellent experience in organization and working with the elderly. Be patient with your instructors. They also are more specialized in some areas than others. Find out more about your instructors' specialties. Try to attend some of the seminars and workshops put on by nursing specialty groups. We don't want you to specialize too soon but there is lots to learn from those who are specialized.

THE CIRCLE OF LEARNING

Fortunately, nursing practica are never solo activities. We like to think of the many people formally and informally involved in clinical rotations as a "circle of learning."

Your Classmates

We put your classmates first because in some ways they are the most important in your circle of learning. Together you will share the anxieties, the thrills, the embarrassing moments, and all that goes into learning the practice of nursing. More than anyone else they will help you to learn to laugh at yourself, to keep your anxieties in check, and to have fun along the way. Exchange phone numbers as soon as you get into your practicum group. Arrange to meet after clinical for coffee. Share articles and drug cards.

Your Practicum Instructor

Your practica instructors have been selected for your nursing education program because they have special skills and knowledge, and the ability to communicate with nursing students. They will be experienced nurses with a particular interest in applied teaching and clinical practice. Nursing experience and advanced educational preparation then are requisites for instructor expertise in order to make the interpretations of nursing practice meaningful to you as a beginning nurse. Your instructors will assist you in learning nursing skills, building your confidence, and meeting the day-to-day challenges of your clinical rotation. They also will assess and evaluate your performance.

Nursing students are accountable to their practica instructors in several ways. You are accountable to the organization in which you are doing your clinical rotation, to your clients, and the nursing profession. Practice safety and quality, professional behavior, and the acquisition of knowledge are expectations vested in you. You are responsible to your instructors to meet these practice expectations. This means that both of you are accountable to the clinical setting for the work you do as well as to your nursing education program.

Power and influence also flow from your practica instructors' expertise and skills as experienced nurses and instructors. As professional nurses in a clinical setting, your instructors may be responsible for the clients with whom you are working or that accountability may be shared with a registered nurse or other health-care provider from the agency or institution. As experienced nurses, they will offer guidance regarding specific client or practice skill problems. As instructors for your nursing education program, they have authority to determine practice assignments. Often this is done in conjunction with you and/or with agency staff, but ultimately it is your instructors' judgements that will prevail as to the complexity of client assignment appropriate for your stage of learning. They evaluate your performance, progress, and learning. You can anticipate that your practica instructors will expect you to get and seek help from them on a regular and frequent basis to ensure your practice is accountable and responsible in all facets of your developing professional skills, knowledge and behaviors. Your clinical rotation instructors are such an important part of your circle of learning that we have devoted a major part of Chapter 5 to discussing this relationship.

Your Practicum Coordinator

Usually there are several instructors and clinical rotation groups in clinical courses. It is the practicum coordinator (sometimes called the course coordinator or the course professor) who is responsible for the overall course. He or she may give an introductory class, distribute the course outline, etc. Your first line of communication for concerns is always your instructor, but if you and your instructor have been unable to resolve an issue then you may need to go to the practicum coordinator. If you have not yet been assigned an instructor but need to discuss something related to the clinical rotation, then you should contact the coordinator.

Your Tutorial Leader

Sometimes you will have a tutorial in conjunction with a clinical practicum. The tutorial leader may be your clinical rotation instructor or, especially if groups are combined, it may a different instructor. We have designed the instructions that go with the learning exercises in each chapter to include a section for tutorial leaders. Sometimes you will be responsible for leading a tutorial and so those ideas might be helpful to you too.

Agency Staff

The relationships you develop with agency staff are an important and often challenging part of clinical practica. To them you may be part of another group of students who they see come and go. Basic principles of courtesy, respect, and recognition of their many responsibilities are important in establishing good relationships. Introduce yourself. Be clear on what you can and cannot do—when you will be coming, how long you will be staying, and so on. Keep agency staff informed about changes in client circumstances. Consult with them. Remember that you leave after a few hours, a shift, a term, but they will continue to carry responsibility for their clients. Most agency staff enjoy working with students and find your questions stimulating. However you do need to be sensitive to their time constraints and other responsibilities. Be helpful where you can.

Collaboration

Collaboration is an underlying theme in nursing education and practice. You may have the opportunity to participate in team conferences as another element to your learning. Team conferences are usually collaborative in nature, and are unique and dynamic opportunities for you to present a nursing perspective about a client or issue. Other peers or professionals may also offer advice or expertise about cases and practice issues, special content, training, or knowledge in an area. Collaboration is a special form of developing accountable and responsible practice for clients.

Clients/Patients

Some of your best teachers will be the clients or patients with whom you work. They are the experts when it comes to living with their particular health risks and problems. From them you will learn what it is like to live with illness or disability, why it is hard to make healthy lifestyle choices, what can make life a little easier in spite of limitations, and about strength, hardiness, and resiliency. Most people like to talk about their situation. Questions like "when did you first realize that you had this health problem? what is it like to have. . . ? what has helped you cope with. . . ?" will unlock a wealth of knowledge. You will find that things you have learned from "experienced" clients/patients will help you understand the actual experience of illness; remember information about signs, symptoms, and treatments; and teach others about managing similar challenges.

Others in Your Life

Friends, families, spouses, and partners are also important to your circle of learning. They can help you balance your life, keep you grounded, and sometimes offer helpful perspectives to dilemmas you may face. Remember, however, the importance of maintaining confidentiality at all times. There will be many situations about which you cannot talk at all. On the other hand, fundamental experiences—seeing your first birth, facing sudden death, feeling overwhelmed with human suffering— are all things that you may find helpful to talk through with the people close to you.

It helps to be clear with family and friends about your needs with respect to each clinical rotation. You might need to remind your spouse that inviting friends over the night before your clinical is not helpful, but that it would be a great way to wind down the night after clinical.

You, the Student

You are the key player in your circle of learning. Nursing practica involve intensive interactions with people. Sometimes you will need to draw away from others, to have time for yourself. Taking care of your needs for sleep, exercise, good nutrition, relaxation, and spiritual renewal is part of ensuring that the key player in your circle of learning is ready for the next challenge (see Chapter 4 for some tips on self-care).

SUMMARY

In this introductory chapter we have looked at different types of clinical rotation formats and overviewed many of the processes involved. The exercises that follow will help you think more deeply about what you expect and bring to your clinical practica. The chapters that follow elaborate most of the ideas introduced in this first chapter. Pick and choose the tools that fit your particular situation. You will find yourself revisiting certain portions over and over. This is *your* workbook. Use it to make notes to yourself, to record your journey, and to chronicle your growth. By so doing you will be able to look back on your journey, each clinical rotation, to see where you have grown and changed. Have fun!

LEARNING TOOL 1.1

Seeing Myself in Clinical Experiences

LEARNING FOCUS: Values Exploration

This exercise gives you an opportunity to examine your feelings about being a nursing student within one of the four clinical formats suggested in this book—observation, instructor-led, preceptored, or internship.

STUDENT ACTION

Choose one type of practicum, perhaps the one that you are currently in or your next clinical experience.

1. List the feelings you have when you think about being in this or your next clinical experience (nervous, excited, insecure, anxious, etc.).

2. Rate the intensity of each feeling listed from 0 to 100 percent. For example, "hardly anxious" might be rated as 20 percent, whereas "very, very anxious" might be 99 percent.

3. Think carefully about some of the cognitive sources of these feelings. Identify at least one attitude, belief, knowledge, or concern that supports or maintains each of these feelings. For example, you might be feeling 88 percent determined and this is supported by the knowledge that "I've made it through all of these years of school and been successful." On the other hand, you might also be feeling 100 percent nervous which is maintained by the attitude "Getting good grades in course work is one thing but putting it all into practice is quite another matter." I don't even know where to start in organizing myself."

4. Are any of these thoughts unrealistic? For example, you might be overgeneralizing things by thinking that you will *never* keep the myriad pieces of information about your cases straight. A more realistic thought would be to remember all of the times you have retained lots of information, such as for exams. Remind yourself. For each unrealistic thought or belief, write a more realistic statement.

Use this example to help you get started:

1. Feeling: *Nervous*

2. Intensity Rating for Feeling: *100%*

3. Concerns, Attitudes, and Beliefs That Maintain the Feeling: *Getting good grades in course work is one thing but putting it all into practice is quite another matter. I don't even know where to start in organizing myself for this.*

4. More Realistic Thought: *This is a learning experience and I'm not expected to know everything. The clinical rotation is about discovering what I do and do not know through trying things in real-life experiences.*

MYSELF IN A _____ PRACTICUM

(Type of Practicum)

1. Feeling:

2. Intensity Rating for Feeling:

3. Concerns, Attitudes, and Beliefs That Maintain the Feeling:

4. More Realistic Thought:

MYSELF IN A _____ **PRACTICUM**

(Type of Practicum)

1. Feeling:

2. Intensity Rating for Feeling:

3. Concerns, Attitudes, and Beliefs That Maintain the Feeling:

4. More Realistic Thought:

MYSELF IN A _____ PRACTICUM
(Type of Practicum)

1. Feeling:

2. Intensity Rating for Feeling:

3. Concerns, Attitudes, and Beliefs That Maintain the Feeling:

4. More Realistic Thought:

MYSELF IN A _____ PRACTICUM
(Type of Practicum)

1. Feeling:

2. Intensity Rating for Feeling:

3. Concerns, Attitudes, and Beliefs That Maintain the Feeling:

4. More Realistic Thought:

NOTES ON USE

Student Use   As you do this and other exercises, remember that your ability and resourcefulness have brought you to this phase in your learning. It is from this place of strength that you should approach all of the work set forth in this handbook. It is a tool to help you deepen and enrich your journey to becoming an effective nurse. The thoughts that maintain your feelings can play an important role in many situations. The process for exploring your thoughts and feelings used in this exercise can be applied in any situation to change the intensity of many feelings. You may use this technique with clients/patients when their feelings are intense. Within the context of theory, this exercise represents a cognitive restructuring technique.

Now try seeing yourself in the other three practicum formats. Just repeat the four steps used above, applying them to the other practicum situations. Then answer these summary questions: In which practicum did you have the strongest confidence-related feelings? In which practicum did you have the strongest anxiety-related feelings? Were there common thoughts maintaining your feelings?

Instructor Use   Some of the student concerns raised during this exercise may be somewhat relieved with more information about the various practica. This might be an appropriate place to draw upon the experiences of former students, who have recently completed some of these practica. You might assign current students to interview the experienced students and gather their stories in written, audio, or video formats. Have students bring these stories to the next tutorial and share them with the group.

You could use the same analysis process (i.e., identify feelings; rate their intensity; identify thoughts, concerns, or attitudes that support or maintain the feelings; and identify more realistic thoughts) in almost any circumstance where feelings are likely to be intense. This will help students to explore and challenge their feelings and thoughts about novel learning situations.

LEARNING TOOL 1.2

Your Circle of Learning and Beyond

LEARNING FOCUS: Knowledge Building

This exercise will provide you with an overview of the persons and groups who form the context of your learning circle and life environment as well as the quality of the relationships. It is designed to help you remember that you live in a dynamic environment.

STUDENT ACTION

Your circle of learning can be illustrated as a picture of your universe with you at the center. Your galaxy includes yourself in relationship to other persons and groups—classmates, clinical instructor, and tutorial leader, as well as others in your life.

1. Create a diagram, or "ecomap," to depict your galaxy. Using Figure 1-1, put yourself in the center of the diagram. Derived from family systems theory, the ecomap is a standard assessment tool used in many nursing contexts. Wright and Leahey (1994) suggest that the outer spheres represent significant people, agencies, and institutions within your context. They suggest that the sizes of the spheres are not important. With this in mind, add as many orbiting spheres as you need to represent the important relationships in your professional life. For example, one sphere will be for your classmates, however, you may want a separate sphere for a classmate with whom you spend a lot of time. Describe how each relationship in your professional and learning spheres acts as a resource or perhaps a stressor for you.

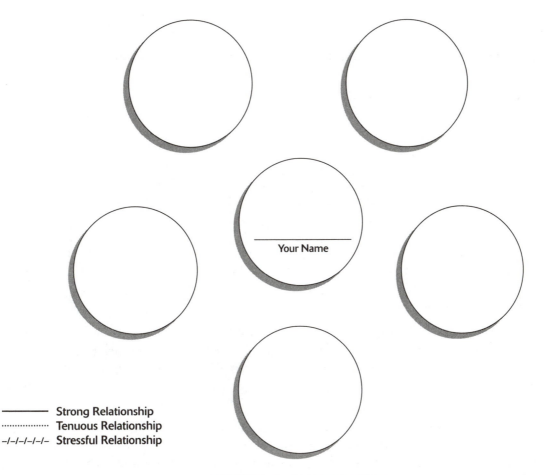

Your Name

——————— Strong Relationship
················· Tenuous Relationship
–/–/–/–/– Stressful Relationship

FIGURE 1–1   My Learning Galaxy

LEARNING TOOL 1.2 continued

2. Now indicate the nature of the connections between yourself and the other spheres with a descriptive word or by drawing different kinds of lines or colored lines. Wright and Leahey suggest that straight lines represent strong connections, whereas dotted and slashed lines represent tenuous and stressful relationships respectively. You could add color for additional visual impact. For example, you may use a solid, green line for strong; a yellow dotted line for tenuous; and a red, slashed line for stressful relationships. The flow of energy can be indicated using arrows. For example, if you get as much energy from a classmate as you give, arrows in both directions would represent this mutual energy flow.

3. Now add other persons, such as family and friends, to your ecomap. These are important members of your learning galaxy. How do each of your family and friend relationships act as a resource or stressor?

Consider your relationships with each of the persons and groups on your ecomap when answering the following questions.

1. Are there classmates with whom you would particularly like to work or not like to work? Identify the reasons for your choices.

2. How would you like to change your relationship with any of the spheres in your galaxy? In what ways could this be accomplished?

NOTES ON USE

Student Use.   Knowing the members of your learning circle will help you to keep things in perspective concerning your relational resources and stressors. Having a dynamic environment means that it will enrich you but each of these resources will also create demands on your time and attention. Your challenge will be to balance the demand and the resource aspects of relationships. Talk with others and see how they keep the balancing act going. That's using relationships as resources!

Instructor Use.   This exercise uses a variation of an assessment mapping tool, the ecomap. An ecomap also will be used in a clinical application as part of Learning Tool 1.4. Later in this book, we will introduce the use of a genogram. It may be helpful for students to have a formal review of these and other mapping techniques. Wright and Leahey (1994) provide an excellent review of these techniques.

LEARNING TOOL 1.3

Myths of a Helping Profession

LEARNING FOCUS: Clinical Thinking Development

In this chapter you explored myths about practicum learning (i.e., Your Practicum Is Not . . .), now you have an opportunity to look at some myths about helping. To manage your clinical nursing experiences successfully, you may want to examine notions that might perpetuate myths about persons in helping professions. These myths may influence how you make decisions.

STUDENT ACTION

Use Myth 1 in the Some Myths of Helping section to guide you in examining your own examples.

1. Identify four myths that you recognize about nursing as a helping profession. You may identify these myths through common stereotypes about nursing, such as the one given in Myth 1.

2. Rate from 0 to 100 percent how strongly you believe in this myth.

3. Myths contain an element of truth. Identify the element of truth in the myth.

4. Write out several examples of when you would use this kernel of truth and when you would not.

SOME MYTHS OF HELPING

Myth 1: Nurses should always be kind and gentle because the client is in some sort of pain.

I believe in this myth _____ %.

The kernel of truth is . . .

I would or would not use this kernel of truth in the following situations.

Myth 2:

I believe in this myth _____ %.

The kernel of truth is . . .

I would or would not use this kernel of truth in the following situations.

Myth 3:

I believe in this myth _____ %.

The kernel of truth is . . .

I would or would not use this kernel of truth in the following situations.

Myth 4:

I believe in this myth _____ %.

The kernel of truth is . . .

I would or would not use this kernel of truth in the following situations.

Myth 5:

I believe in this myth _____ %.

The kernel of truth is . . .

I would or would not use this kernel of truth in the following situations.

NOTES ON USE

Student Use.   As you complete this and other exercises, pay attention to those exercises that you enjoy more than others or for which you find the structure of the exercise more to your liking. In future chapters, we will talk about preferred ways of learning. Your responses to these early exercises may help you discover your preferred ways of learning. Preferred learning information can be helpful in understanding why you learn better in some circumstances or ways.

Instructor Use.   The sections in "Your Practicum is Not . . ." are a type of demythologizing. This demythologizing is extended in this exercise by exploring the myths of helping. There are hidden expectations behind these myths and this exercise will help students uncover these expectations about the nursing profession. The demythologizing process can be expanded to include myths about the helping settings (e.g., hospital, community settings) as well as about being a student nurse.

This exercise can produce fruitful small and/or large group discussions. Your class can also create a master list of myths. Encourage students to update the list and give examples from their clinical experiences. The exercise could be extended to include how these prevalent myths are perpetuated in the profession as well as how they affect the expectations of clients/patients.

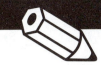

LEARNING TOOL 1.4

Client Context

LEARNING FOCUS: Application Enhancement

You have been considering your context of learning throughout this chapter. Now we would like you to apply your learning to thinking about the importance of context for patients/clients. The focus of this exercise is to apply context awareness to a case example.

STUDENT ACTION

As a nursing student your work context will change from clinical rotation to clinical rotation. You may find yourself in nursing contexts such as hospitals, nursing homes, and community agencies. Here is a case example from a nursing home context:

> *Mrs. Romero is an elderly woman. She seems withdrawn and appears to not want to talk. Mrs. Romero doesn't want to be here. She is hemiplegic from a stroke four years ago. Her family visits her every Sunday after Mass. They mostly speak to her in Italian. Once a month, the priest comes to give her communion. Otherwise, she rarely has visitors. Her roommate, Mrs. Kolenski, has some cognitive impairment but is more physically mobile. However, in the past she has accused Mrs. Romero of stealing things from her.*

1. Develop an ecomap for Mrs. Romero. An ecomap is a diagram of a person's environmental resources and constraints—necessary knowledge for designing and implementing solutions—and represents the important individuals and groups with whom a person interacts. Using Figure 1-2, put Mrs. Romero in the center of the ecomap. Then use the outer spheres to represent significant people, agencies, and institutions within Mrs. Romero's environment. As Wright and Leahey (1994) suggest, the size of the spheres is not important. With this in mind, add as many spheres as you need to represent Mrs. Romero's important relationships. Remember to include the quality of relationship between Mrs. Romero and the individuals, groups, and institutions involved. Include yourself and other health care professionals who would be involved with Mrs. Romero.

MRS. ROMERO'S ECOMAP

Use this diagram to help you get started with the ecomap.

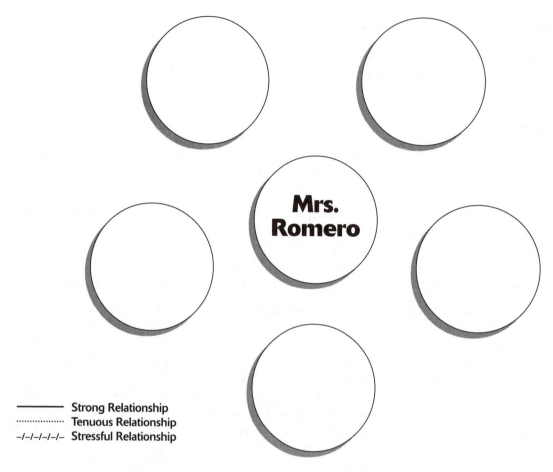

─────── Strong Relationship
··············· Tenuous Relationship
–/–/–/–/– Stressful Relationship

FIGURE 1–2 Mrs. Romero's Ecomap

2. Describe how each of the relationships in Mrs. Romero's life may act as a resource or perhaps as a stressor.

3. What changes would you need to make to the ecomap if you were encountering Mrs. Romero in a different context, such as a hospital unit or community agency?

4. Using the context-related information given, discuss how you would use this information to develop and implement care planning for Mrs. Romero?

NOTES ON USE

Student Use. Derived from family systems theory, the ecomap is a standard assessment tool used in many nursing contexts. Like other exercises, this learning tool is intended to get you thinking about nursing activities and exploring them from a personal as well as a nursing perspective. You might find it enriching to compare your answers with those of other classmates. Remember, there are no right and wrong answers. Your comparisons are to expand your learning. Others will have new ways for you to look at things. After you share with others, write down things that you would now change about your case reflections. This means applying new information to modify your ideas—a very important skill!

Instructor Use. You can use this exercise with dyads during postconference sessions. If they are completing this as a dyad, have the students reflect on what new perspectives the other student brought to their own way of thinking about the case. You might point out how this may reflect a person's preferred way of learning (see Chapter 5 for details about the learning styles reviewed in this book). For example, the "converger" learning style may experience frustration with the no right answer aspect of the case, while the student with an "assimilator" learning style will likely add a lot of detail to the exercise. To help students appreciate their unique contributions and thinking, you might explore how different or alike are the approaches of the students in the dyads or what the dyads share with the whole group. You could also explore how students feel about the differences, which is especially helpful for students with a "diverger" learning style. This will encourage feeling awareness associated with differences, as well as how student nurses are unique in their thinking and feeling.

LEARNING TOOL 1.5

Keeping a Journal

JOURNAL FOCUS

Every journal is unique and personal. Your nursing student journal will take shape as you develop as a nurse. You will discover important ways on your own to express yourself. The important thing as you write in your journal is to keep looking for what is more meaningful and more central to you, for the influences that shape the events and the patterns of your life as a nursing student.

Journal writing is different from keeping a diary in that the latter is primarily guided by external events and the former is directed more at internal themes. Although outer events may be recorded, the purpose of writing about them is to reflect upon their meaning for your inner life. That is, you become more aware of the significance of these events in regard to your inner processes. The focus will be on your unfolding awareness of yourself and your world, as well as the new meanings, values, and interrelationships you are discovering. (For more detailed information see Chapter 6—Logging Life's Ups and Downs.)

STUDENT ACTION

This journal writing exercise promotes emotional awareness and, perhaps, catharsis. Describe a situation from your clinical experience that was highly emotionally charged—positively or negatively. Here are two actual entries from student journals to spark your reflection.

> I have to be honest. I was really nervous about going to a nursing home even though I have had some experience with the elderly. I imagined the nursing home to be like the home in the article we read in class, "Can the clinical milieu be therapeutic," in which the rooms were dark and residents were terrorized instead of cared for. But I must admit, the surroundings eased my discomfort when I got there. It was one of the many pleasant experiences I've had so far.
>
> In the mental health area, we deal with patients who tend to have emotional and mental pain, instead of physical pain. I realize, in the holistic view, that this is really all the same. Sometimes, I feel like I have emotional and mental pain when dealing with stresses of my own.

1. Describe your own emotionally charged experience in some detail—mention the who, what, when, where, and why. Use your observation skills to help you recall not only the essence but the particulars as well.

2. What was it like emotionally to be part of this experience?

3. Did you play a central role in the situation or a more peripheral role?

4. How did you feel about your emotional responses?

5. Would you like something of your emotional response to be different? Why or why not?

6. How might things have been different if you were able to respond differently?

7. Write about an experience in which you did respond in your more preferred way.

8. What did you learn from this situation that may help you in another highly charged situation in the future?

POSITIVE STATEMENTS ABOUT ME

This section of your journal is to draw out from your reflections and journal writing positive statements you can make about yourself. When we focus on our learning, it is very easy to forget about what we already know, think, and do. This section gives you an opportunity to pay attention to these aspects of yourself. Make each statement an "I" statement. For example, "I felt proud that I asked my instructor the question about . . ." or "I was able to help my client feel more comfortable by . . ."

NOTES ON USE

Student Use.   You may have already had a lot of experience with journal writing. If this is true, then adapt this exercise to suit your needs. One suggestion is that you reflect back to the time when you were beginning and look at how you would address that experience from where you now are. When you explore situations with this kind of detail and investigation, you create important memories about what you learned from specific cases. These cases can become "paradigm cases"—clinical experiences that alter your way of seeing future situations. You may want to create a special section for paradigm cases or find a way to tag paradigm cases from within the text of your journal writing. Be creative!

Instructor Use.   It may be helpful for you to direct a discussion about how the journal exercises in this book can complement your own use of journaling assignments. You are the primary person responsible for the journaling experiences of your students, so use these exercises to supplement your own. We have found that collecting some journal entries, and perhaps publishing them in a newsletter, can be a wonderful way of sharing experiences among students. These can help to normalize the experiences of the novice nursing student.

CHAPTER

2

Ethics and Dilemmas

JOURNAL THOUGHT

Nursing has really allowed me the ability to experience my own education firsthand and let me question my morals, values, and ethics. It is a complete mixture of science and humanity . . . I am looking forward to the years ahead with anticipation and confidence. I am aware there are many obstacles to overcome, but the journey should be one to remember.

NURSING STUDENT

ETHICS AND DILEMMAS

There will be many places in your nursing program where you learn about ethics. You may have been introduced to your national nursing association's code of ethics in your first nursing course. You may be required or have the option to take a course on ethics during your nursing program. You may have taken part in values clarification exercises or engaged in discussions on specific ethical/moral issues. You can draw also on your personal life experience, cultural background, spiritual values, what you have read and seen in the media on high profile ethical issues, and your personal struggles and dilemmas.

It is one thing to talk about ethical issues but clinical practice puts you into situations where you are frequently challenged by real-life dilemmas and the need to make ethical decisions. The high value that nurses put on client/patient advocacy is essentially an ethical stance. Because of this stance, simple decisions such as whether to put in a second call to a physician because a patient is insisting he needs something more for his pain can be seen as examples of ethical decision making. Nor is such a seemingly simple decision all that easy when put into context. It would seem that advocating for the client's need would clearly be the guiding principle.

This example came from the experience of a nursing student in a preceptored practicum during the final year of her program. The situation occurred in a rural community where there was only one physician available, and he had left the hospital to see other patients in the town clinic. Although the nursing student did not think of the concept at that moment, part of the dilemma she was experiencing was related to the ethical principle of justice. In other words, what was fair and equitable given competing patient needs? At the time the student nurse's preceptor gave her some practical advice on handling the situation with the patient and the physician (important clinical learning also). After her shift, however, she reflected in her journal that she was still struggling with the dilemma. Later as she and her instructor explored the situation together they saw it for its ethical significance, which gave her a new way of thinking about handling similar situations in the future.

This chapter will help you begin to recognize and consider some of the ethical issues that you will experience in clinical practice—how to prepare for them and to maximize the ethical learning opportunities they present.

CLIENT/PATIENT–RELATED ETHICAL ISSUES

It seems like a paradox but the first step in dealing with client-related issues is to understand your own values as well as how those values may be triggered by clinical situations. The second step is learning to recognize situations, like the one discussed in the preceding example, that have ethical implications. The third step is to seek out help in reflecting on the dilemmas that confront you. Individual or group meetings with your instructor are ideal times for such explorations, as is journaling.

Some clinical situations may be particularly troubling, globally or individually. Global issues are the ethical dilemmas that face society in general: end-of-life decisions, allocation of scarce resources, the possibilities of genetic manipulation, and so on. Faced with knowing that tomorrow you will be caring for a severely brain-injured fourteen-year-old girl whose parents and physicians have decided should no longer receive tube feedings because of her persistent vegetative state transforms a global issue into a very personal one. On one hand, you may respect the right of the parents to make this decision. On the other hand, you may be feeling very troubled about being part of this young girl's care when to you caring is about providing, not withholding.

Other clinical situations may bring you into conflict with your moral or religious values. If you anticipate or encounter such a problem, discuss it with your clinical instructor who can guide you with respect to your rights as well as those of the client. Few situations are black and white. To you it may be morally wrong to have an abortion, but does that make it morally wrong for you to provide nursing care for someone who has made a different choice? Is there a difference between actually administering a "morning after" pill versus listing it as one of the alternatives that a young woman might consider?

Most situations involving ethical dilemmas are less dramatic but no less important:

- resisting the urge to talk about what just happened on the unit while riding down to lunch on the public elevator;
- seeing a personal care aide slap an aggressive elderly patient with dementia;
- having a clinic patient confide in you that she does not want to take part in the clinical trial but she is afraid that her doctor will be angry with her if she does not; or
- finding out that the health-care agency is using funds, raised through a major campaign for handicapped children, primarily to support services for adults "because people give more if they think it is for children."

Notes

You are responsible, even as a nursing student, to know and practice your professional code of ethics. We have provided excerpts from the codes of the International Council of Nursing, the American Nurses Association, and the Canadian Nurses Association in the Appendix. Read (or reread) them now so that what they say comes to your mind easily when you are confronted by ethical dilemmas.

CLINICAL LEARNING–RELATED ETHICAL ISSUES

The types of situations discussed up to now occur whether or not you are a nursing student. But there are other types of ethical issues that emerge or that might be thought of differently *because* you are a student. For example, all nurses are ethically responsible to maintain their competency and to use judgement in relation to individual competence when accepting and delegating responsibilities. Right now you may wonder if you are really competent at anything. During much of your clinical practica, you will be encountering skills that you are doing for the first time or that you may have only done once or twice before. You are learning to become competent, but your skill set is developing and is greatly affected by whether you have had certain opportunities. Even your instructor may need to rely in part on your judgement as to whether you are competent to handle a particular procedure or situation alone. Therefore, it is your responsibility to seek out supervision if you:

- have not done a procedure before;
- do not feel confident that you are ready to do it without supervision;
- have never done the procedure with this type of client (e.g., giving an injection to a child or doing an assessment interview with a suicidal adolescent);
- have been having problems doing the procedure (e.g., changing a complex intravenous setup); or
- know that there is a high risk for the client and/or that the procedure requires particular qualifications (e.g., you may have excellent skills starting IVs under supervision but the institutional policy states that only registered nurses can do that procedure).

Accountability for what you do or have forgotten to do is an ethical expectation of nursing students (and graduates) at any level. We realize that students make mistakes and that is part of learning. However, in our profession client safety is a major issue. Therefore, part of your education is learning how to be accountable in the context of nursing practice. Many of you already have a highly developed sense of accountability. For you it is important to recognize what warrants reporting versus what does not need to be reported but for which you are accountable. For example, being ten minutes late in administering a once-a-day medication does not warrant reporting. The overly conscientious student may need to learn to not bother an instructor or staff nurse with that information but if asked should be honest about the time it was given. On the other hand, some of you may feel that you have survived to this point by not acknowledging your errors of commission or omission. Not having done the required readings for class is one thing, but trying to bluff your way through the action of the medication you are about to give is quite another. A straightforward "I don't know" will do much more for your survival in nursing. Clinical instructors develop a fairly high tolerance for mistakes but an incident of dishonesty or lack of accountability can jeopardize your career.

Other ethical issues relate to personal conduct. Taking medication from the agency is not ethically appropriate even if you do develop a migraine while you are there. Gossiping is likewise unacceptable. Sometimes it is hard to decide what is gossiping and what is blowing off steam. It is okay to vent your frustrations with a close friend; it is not okay to start a rumor about the unfairness of a particular instructor.

In nursing practica you are often in emotionally intense situations with your instructor, peers, clients and families, or other health providers. It is easy for the boundaries between personal and professional relationships to blur. What if a client asks you out for dinner, or a deceased patient's family gives you an expensive gift? Your nursing program may have guidelines for such situations. If not, discuss them with your instructor.

ਟੇ SUMMARY

You will encounter many ethical issues and dilemmas in your clinical rotations. Just as there are tools to help you with other elements of clinical learning so there are tools to help you deal with ethical issues. One set of tools, the codes of ethics of our profession, gives us direction in terms of caring, autonomy, respecting human dignity, confidentiality, accountability, and competence. Another set of tools is knowledge of personal values and the influences that culture and beliefs have on those values. Knowing ethical principles and practicing them in clinical situations is another tool. Reflecting on your practice and the dilemmas you face through journaling and interacting with your instructor and classmates is another valuable tool.

LEARNING TOOL 2.1

Would You Believe?

LEARNING FOCUS: Values Exploration

Your beliefs and expectations influence your reactions to clients and patients. These beliefs and expectations may be about several aspects of the patient/client and their situation. This exercise will give you a chance to examine some of your own expectations and beliefs.

STUDENT ACTION

Directions are included in each section.

1. Imagine that you are very depressed and confused. Your partner is taking you to the local health clinic. Describe your thoughts and feelings.

Complete the following sentences:

People who have a mental illness are . . .

Helping people who have a mental illness is . . .

2. Did you ever seek help for a serious medical problem? If yes, what were your feelings at the time? If you have never been in this situation, talk with someone you know. Write about the feelings he or she experienced.

3. When you need advice or have a problem, to whom do you turn for help? Give three examples, and explain why you would confer with this person.

4. Complete the following sentences. They will help you examine your personal beliefs concerning some frequently encountered situations.

   Abortion is . . .

   People who have abortions are usually . . .

People over seventy are usually . . .

If an elderly relative wanted to live with me, I would . . .

5. Describe one way in which you are or feel "different" from others that you are ready and willing to discuss. The difference may be a cultural or ethnic one, or perhaps some physical or emotional aspect of your self, or even some religious belief or custom. How has this affected your life?

NOTES ON USE

Student Use.   This exercise challenges you to get personal because it examines some very private thoughts and beliefs. There are no right or wrong answers to these questions or sentence completions. Be honest with yourself but remember that you can decide what you wish to share with others. This exercise may provoke concerns about being judged for what you believe. People are different and this is as true for you as nursing students as it will be for your clients/patients. Practicing tolerance with your classmates may be challenging but will bear fruit in your clinical rotation experiences. Expect that you will be accepted for who you are. Though you will not want to change beliefs that are fundamental to who you are, realize that you may want to change some beliefs and expectations once you have articulated them more clearly. Coming to terms with these distinctions will put you in better stead for the experiences you will face in the future.

Instructor Use.   Self-awareness is the focus of many exercises throughout this handbook. These exercises can complement your teaching and provide opportunities for you to give positive, honest feedback to students. You can provide the link between beliefs and values and their impact on clients/patients. As you know, this linking of personal and professional is crucial in the development of your students' professional identities. You are a major socialization agent in the development of your students' professional identities.

This exercise may be particularly sensitive and personal for students. Your judgement as to how much of this exercise you will invite them to share in a group setting will depend upon the level of trust and cohesiveness of the group, the time available, and what you want to bring out in relation to their current clinical context. You may want to take the lead in sharing how a value of yours has changed or not changed over time and how it may have affected your practice. One of your "paradigm cases" may be an excellent example for this discussion.

LEARNING TOOL 2.2

Getting at the Roots

LEARNING FOCUS: Knowledge Building

Many of our beliefs, values, and expectations of helping and other issues come from our cultural experience. This exercise is designed to help you explore your cultural heritage and experience. You will be asked to develop a cultural genogram. A genogram is like a family tree and a cultural genogram is a family tree with cultural information added to it.

STUDENT ACTION

1. Place yourself at the bottom of the genogram in Figure 2-1. Convention dictates using circles for females and squares for males. Put your name and age inside the square or circle. You may want to write several words that describe personal qualities and/or things you enjoy doing beside your square or circle.

2. Family members are placed on horizontal rows representing each generation (Wright & Leahey, 1994). Now place any older siblings to the left of you and younger siblings to the right in squares/circles along the horizontal line. Place a sibling's name and age in each figure. If any sibling is deceased, place an *X* through it and insert the year of death within the circle or square.

3. Your parents are represented in the generation line just above yours. Vertical lines connect you and any siblings to your parents' generation horizontal line. Indicate along the horizontal line that joins your mother and father how long they have been married. If your parents are divorced put two small slashes (//) through the line that joins them and the year of the divorce or separation.

4. Develop the genogram of your family of origin going back to the first generation that came to the country in which you now reside, if you can.

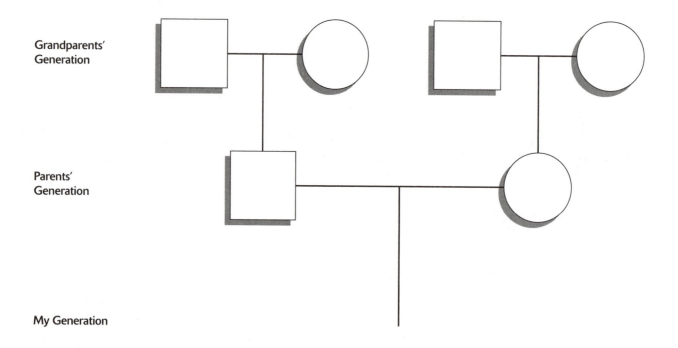

FIGURE 2-1   Cultural Genogram

5. After drawing the generations, indicate the ethnic and cultural roots of each person. You may need to draw upon sources beyond your personal knowledge, such as parents, grandparents, and other relatives or literary resources. Create a "legend" for the cultures represented on your genogram. You might want to designate different ethnic heritages by using different designs and colors within the circles and squares. For example, green might represent an Irish heritage or a tartan a Scottish ancestry.

Answer the following questions to further explore your cultural and ethnic roots.

1. What are the major group(s) from which you are descended?

2. From whom did you learn about your ethnic background?

3. What shaped the beliefs and behaviors of your cultures of origin (consider cultural beliefs about own and other cultures, role of rituals and religion, time of migration, place of family, etc.)?

LEARNING TOOL 2.2 continued

4. What ethnic or cultural characteristics were purposefully suppressed, concealed, or disapproved of in your family (e.g., dropping out of school, certain medical or mental health conditions, etc.)?

5. What characteristics were sources of pride within your culture (e.g., education, family wealth, etc.)?

NOTES ON USE

Student Use.   Have fun with this exercise. Here is a time to tap some of those resource relationships you identified in the previous chapter's exercises. You may even get family members interested in your project. It's great when you can involve them in what you are doing. You might even want to "publish" your findings throughout your family and have them add any information that you missed. In the end you could give your "roots" genogram to family members—what a great gift for future generations too! Remember, knowing your own heritage is the starting point for raising your cultural awareness and increasing your cultural sensitivity.

Instructor Use.   You could use a cultural genogram to explore the history and values of the nursing profession. Look at the historical roots of nursing and the cultural context in which the profession emerged and developed. You can also create a cultural genogram on a smaller scale for the agency in which the students are practicing. Comparing cultural genograms for public and private institutions as well as secular and religious organizations can help students gain greater appreciation for how these agencies handle certain ethical dilemmas.

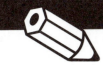

LEARNING TOOL 2.3

Making the Connections

LEARNING FOCUS: Critical Thinking Development

Thinking critically about beliefs, values, and expectations means raising questions about all kinds of views that you hold. Different cultural and ethnic experiences create unique ways of viewing self, others and the world.

STUDENT ACTION

Use the information you gained in doing the previous exercise on developing a cultural genogram to examine the following assumptions and classifications. Later you will be asked to explore the assumptions and beliefs in terms of their potential consequences for effective nursing practice.

    Complete the first sentence of each of the following pairs from the traditional perspective within your ethnic and cultural experience. Complete the second sentence based on your personal views that *may* or *may not* differ from the traditional norms written about in the first part.

1. Caregiving is believed to be . . .

    I believe caregiving is . . .

2. Women are viewed as . . .

    I view women as . . .

3. Men are assumed to be . . .

I assume men to be . . .

4. Higher education is considered as . . .

I consider higher education as . . .

5. Power and status are . . .

For me, power and status are . . .

6. Homosexuality is seen as . . .

I see homosexuality as . . .

7. Looking different or being a member of another race is viewed as . . .

I view looking different or being a member of another race as . . .

8. Whom one should marry is determined by . . .

I think that whom one should marry is determined by . . .

9. Physical disabilities are assumed to be . . .

I assume physical disabilities to be . . .

10. Personal problems are seen as . . .

I see personal problems as . . .

LEARNING TOOL 2.3 continued

11. Technology is believed to be . . .

    I believe technology to be . . .

12. Medical personnel are held in . . .

    I hold medical personnel in . . .

LEARNING TOOL 2.3 continued

NOTES ON USE

Student Use.   This exercise takes the Learning Tool 2.2 exercise one step further. Here you have a chance to explore the influence of your cultural heritage on your belief system. Remember that clients will have similar influences, so this exercise will sensitize you to their cultural experiences. You might want to discuss with experienced nurses how they have dealt with cultural impacts in their patient care.

Instructor Use.   Using your professional code of ethics, you can extend this exercise by including a discussion of how some of the students' cultural and personal values, beliefs, and biases would be in conflict in a nursing situation. You could then discuss ethical dilemmas that arise from conflicts between personal and professional or between client/patient and professional values, beliefs, or assumptions.

LEARNING TOOL 2.4

Client Values and Caregiving

LEARNING FOCUS: Application Enhancement

In resolving ethical dilemmas, you will need to consider many factors including your personal and professional and patient/client values, beliefs, and expectations. You will also need to consider standards of nursing practice, policies, and procedures of your work environment, and legal statutes in considering an ethical dilemma. The following exercise will give you some practice in applying principles for examining an ethical dilemma.

STUDENT ACTION

Answer the questions following the case example. These questions will help you explore the many dimensions that must be considered in ethical dilemmas.

> *It started in my first year of nursing. We were to interview an elderly person living in the community to find out what health meant to them. She invited me to stay for a cup of tea after the interview. She told me how lonely she felt, that her daughter and grandchildren never had time for her anymore. I listened. When it was time for me to go she pleaded with me to come again. I felt sorry for her and lonely for my own grandmother who lives across the country. I used to stop in after my classes. She would make tea and, on her good days, tell me stories about her early days as a schoolteacher. I started noticing that her memory was failing, that she didn't seem to be eating much. One day she had a bruise on her face but she wouldn't tell me why. I didn't see her for a few weeks. The next time I went there was no answer at the door. Since my current practicum was at the nearest community hospital I managed to check the admission list through the computer. Sure enough she was on one of the medical units. I stopped in to see her after my shift. I still had my uniform and name tag on. At first she didn't recognize me. In fact, I'm not sure if she did remember who I was. But she was crying and pleading with me to help her go home. She seemed to understand that her daughter had arranged for her to go to a nursing home. She had always told me that she'd rather die than be shipped off to the "poorhouse" with "all those crazy people." She asked if I would come and live with her and take care of her. I figured she could afford such an arrangement and wondered why her daughter hadn't thought of that.*

1. What theoretical and factual knowledge do you have that can be applied to your understanding of this situation?

2. What personal values and beliefs do you hold concerning this client/patient and her situation?

3. What ethical principles are relevant to this situation (e.g., respect for persons, beneficence, justice)?

4. How does the nursing code(s) of ethics (see appendices) inform thinking about this situation?

5. Would any ethical guidelines of the hospital or agency be relevant to this situation?

6. What values, beliefs, and expectations of the client/patient system are important to understanding the ethical dilemma?

7. Are any legal regulations relevant to this dilemma?

8. If ethical dilemmas are the result of conflicting values, what competing values are in conflict here?

9. What alternatives are available to you and the patient/client? Identify elements of action plans for each of these alternatives.

10. Identify and weigh the pros and cons of each action plan to both you and the patient/client; then choose what seems to be the most ethical course of action. Give the rationale to support your plan of action.

11. Indicate how much you relied on each of the following sources of information in reaching your ethical "best practice" choice. Choose one of the following four frequency descriptions.

	Not at All	*A Little*	*Somewhat*	*A Great Deal*

Personal critical reflection _____

Discussions with other classmates or peers _____

Nursing literature _____

Discussions with instructor or other experienced nurses _____

The nursing code of ethics _____

Personal value system _____

Discussions with family and friends _____

NOTES ON USE

Student Use. Work with someone else to complete the final two steps of the ethical analysis process. Having the input of another person can help expand your considerations. You may need to begin with a discussion to see if you and your partner have similar or differing personal values. This will affect your agreeing on a "best practice choice."

Instructor Use. Ethical issues may arise from failing to act as well as action options. Have your students describe a situation of omission that has arisen in their clinical placements. Help them to walk through the process of ethical analysis in thinking about that situation. Have them describe the potential consequences of this omission for the persons involved. Talk about what factors could have informed a more appropriate clinical decision. You might encourage students to be alert for incidents such as this in the media that you can use as teaching examples. This case situation may also be used to generate discussion about the everyday decisions students make that have ethical implications (e.g., professional boundaries, confidentiality of health information, etc.).

LEARNING TOOL 2.5

Maxims for Living and Working

JOURNAL FOCUS

We all have maxims—cryptic descriptions of performance—that we use in our daily life. Identifying these can be a skill that you can use in your nursing life as well. Begin by focusing on your personal life.

STUDENT ACTION

1. Identify several maxims that you heard from your parents or other significant persons in your life. They may be in the form of sayings such as "a stitch in time saves nine" or you may have adapted the sayings or maxims into your own words such as "don't do twice what you can do once."

2. Reflect on how these maxims are lived out or might be lived out in your role as a nursing student. Write down these reflections.

3. The following excerpt was part of a reflection of a student nurse after her first month in her first clinical rotation. In her journal writing, she creates a type of maxim by playing with a metaphor and using it to graphically depict her experience.

> *Since September, a new and exciting phenomenon has entered my life. Journaling. In this last four weeks, I have found no time to eat, sleep, or otherwise enjoy the other good things life has to offer. I have single-handedly probed, related, reflected, dug for meaning, and analyzed my concept of health to death. I have written enough to have stripped a forest clean of trees. Clear cut journaling!*

Take the maxim examples you wrote about in the first question and describe how they might relate to nursing situations.

4. You will find or develop helpful maxims for your nursing practice. Keep an ear and an eye open for them. Most often they are short, simple statements that help you to keep on track. "Focus on strengths" and "When in doubt—ask" are two examples that are applicable to both clinical and personal experiences. Write down as many maxims for nursing as you know.

POSITIVE STATEMENTS ABOUT ME

Remember, at the end of each journal entry you are to draw out from your reflections and journal writing positive statements you can make about yourself. Make each statement an "I" statement.

NOTES ON USE

Student Use.   This could be the beginning of a collection of maxims or sayings that are significant to you. As you become more aware of these, you will hear them from patients/clients, from instructors and cleaning staff, from peers and elders. You may want to create a special section in your journal to gather these maxims. Use this section as a quick inspiration when you are finding it difficult to handle a situation.

Instructor Use.   Maxims are described by Benner (1984) as a sort of shorthand used by more experienced nurses to replace the many detailed decision-making rules used by novice learners. Identifying maxims used in their everyday lives and beginning to relate them to nursing will help students maximize their transition from novice to more proficient learner. As an experienced nurse, you can provide many examples of your own use of maxims in professional situations.

PART TWO

Tools for Learning

CHAPTER

3

The Toolbox

JOURNAL THOUGHT

One would think it would be easy to explore yourself, but really it's one of the hardest things to do . . . This program teaches you about caring in every aspect. It lets you understand yourself so that when we go out into the units we can understand how the patients are feeling.

NURSING STUDENT

Why bother with a toolbox? Is it not enough to have the tools? Good questions! In fact, you might want to go after the tools first, in which case you would read Chapter 4 before this one. However, just as a toolbox provides organized and ready access to the tools that may be needed, so this chapter offers practical strategies for overall success.

You might think of your practicum toolbox as having four sides, a top and a bottom (see Figure 3-1). The bottom, that on which everything else rests is the learning process itself. Therefore, we begin this chapter with a section on learning about learning. The four sides can be thought of as your personal resources: feelings, interests, experiences, and capabilities. The top of the toolbox can be thought of as the clinical rotation setting.

Notes

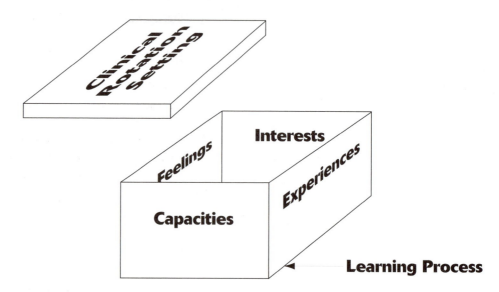

FIGURE 3–1   Your Practicum Toolbox

🔊 LEARNING ABOUT LEARNING

What makes learning easier for you? Do you prefer to read about something new, think about it, and then apply it? Or would you rather learn by doing?

Learning Style Preferences

Studies have shown than the majority of nurses prefer a concrete sequential style. If you like to come out of tutorial with a clear, orderly set of notes, that might be your preferred style. Sometimes you may feel frustrated when an instructor seems to get side-tracked or tries to get a lot of group participation. On the other hand, if you get excited about abstract ideas you might feel a bit bored if your tutorial instructor gives you a list of directions about how to do something in the clinical area. Recognizing these differences can help you maximize your learning experiences, especially in your clinical practica.

Talking to your clinical instructors or preceptors about how you learn best may help them to better understand what you need. For example, you may be able to negotiate an opportunity to observe before doing if that is what works best for you. For more on understanding your learning style and making that work for you see Chapter 5.

Learning-That and Learning-How

Your clinical rotations are contexts for *learning-how*. Your classes and readings are about *learning-that*. These two different kinds of knowledge will gradually become so enmeshed that you will scarcely be able to distinguish them. But, as you start a new practicum, be it your first or your fifth, you will be aware of situations that call for new ways of knowing-how and knowing-that which you have not yet integrated.

Learning-how is most often associated with psychomotor skills but really extends to all aspects of clinical practice. If you are like most nursing students, however, it is uncertainty about the ability to do psychomotor skills that creates much of the anxiety. *Psychomotor* literally means the integration of cognitive and motor functions of the brain. Nursing skills, like other skills you have learned, eventually have their own "motor program" in the brain.

Think of how it was when you first learned to ride a bicycle or drive a car. Each part—starting, stopping, turning a corner—had to be learned and seemed to require your utmost concentration. Then came the modifications of driving on a hill, on a dirt road, and so on. Likewise, taking a client's blood pressure is a complex task and yet it too will become as natural as riding a bicycle or driving a car. But natural does not mean mechanical. As the basics of the skill become more seamless, more of your concentration is available for the client and the unique aspects of each encounter.

Taxonomy of Psychomotor Behavior

Understanding the stages of psychomotor learning can help you set realistic goals for yourself and see your progress (Dave, 1970).

Level of Imitation.   This level involves your first experience with a particular skill after learning the related principles, and seeing pictures or a demonstration of the performance of the skill. You begin practicing the skill by imitating what you have observed and applying what you have read. At this level your performance is expected to be awkward, slow, and nonsequential.

Level of Manipulation.   This level involves overcoming your awkwardness so you can skillfully manipulate the specific pieces of equipment or supplies associated with the skill. It is expected that you will require frequent reference to directions (such as a "performance checklist") in order to execute the skill sequentially. Achieving this level will probably require many repetitions of the skill in the psychomotor skills laboratory. Be patient.

Level of Precision.   At this level you will be able to perform the skill independent of a set of directions, however, you are still expected to be slow. You will probably have to concentrate on each component of the skill, therefore, not allowing much mental space to consider the needs of the involved client.

Level of Articulation.   At this level you can perform the skill with a lesser degree of mental concentration on each small component of the skill, therefore, you are becoming aware of the needs of the involved client. Your actions are deliberate, coordinated, and more efficient. Doing the skill will be less time-consuming.

Level of Naturalization.   At this level your performance of the skill is smooth, natural, and expeditious. You do not have to consciously think about each aspect of the skill, therefore, you can be much more sensitive to the needs of the client. Communication while doing the skill will also become more natural.

Planning to Manage Your Learning

Getting an overall perspective as to what a particular clinical rotation is all about can be very helpful, particularly if getting the big picture first is your preferred way of thinking. Getting down to specifics is also important whether you are a big picture thinker or major on minors. The specifics are what you *need* to know for survival and success. The next two sets of questions will help you zero in on those specifics.

Questions for Your Clinical Instructor.

❧ What do you expect from me? (e.g., care plans, journals, self-evaluation)

❧ What is the best way—phone number(s), beeper, office hours—for me to contact you?

Notes

- What if I am sick? (Who needs to be contacted? How can I get a message through when the office is closed?)
- What skills and client conditions should I review?
- What skills and procedures do you want to watch me do when they first come up in this practicum? (E.g., you may have gotten to the point that you were doing subcutaneous injections without supervision in your last rotation but a new instructor will probably want to spot-check your developing skills)
- Is it okay to be supervised by other staff if you are not readily available?
- What do you think is really important for us to get out of this rotation?
- Do you have any tips? pet peeves?

Questions from Your Clinical Instructor.   Your clinical instructors will probably ask you what your goals are for each practicum. They will usually find it helpful to know where your previous rotations have been and what you see as your strengths and areas to work on. You might be asked about how you learn best, what skills you have and have not done, types of clients with whom you have worked, and so on.

Remember that it will be just as important for your clinical instructor to be able to reach you as vice versa. Instructors usually receive printouts from the registrar's office of students registered in their courses. Therefore, be sure that your educational institution has your current phone number. There may be other numbers that would facilitate communication as well—a beeper number, a work number, your e-mail address. Nothing is more frustrating to instructors than being called at midnight because a student took the narcotics keys home or forgot to chart something, then finding that the only number they have was disconnected last month.

PERSONAL RESOURCES

Your personal resources are the sides of your toolbox. They are part of you as you progress through different practica.

Your Feelings

One of your biggest resources is the caring you feel for others. Focusing on easing their pain can help to allay some of your own anxieties. Other feelings are assets too. Don't be afraid to laugh or cry with clients at times. The genuineness that you bring to situations is part of shared human experience. There will be other times when it is not appropriate to show your feelings; part of your learning is to know which is which.

Your Interests

One of the wonderful things about nursing as a career is its tremendous variability. If you are an avid backpacker you will have learned a lot about self-reliance and have probably sought out some knowledge about wilderness first aid. Do you love music? How might that help you engage a fourteen-year-old or empathize with a professional singer about to have a laryngectomy?

Your Experiences

You have already accumulated a wealth of life experiences. Whether it is your specialized knowledge of a particular sport, your cultural heritage, the chronic illness of a family member, or your worst baby-sitting nightmare you will find that sometime in your nursing career that life experience will come in handy.

Your Capabilities

Are you ambidextrous? Being able to use either hand, and better yet both hands, at the same time, is a great help in psychomotor skills like removing sutures. Do you have a good memory? Are you a good organizer? See the exercises at the end of this chapter for how to do a full inventory of your personal resources.

THE PRACTICUM SETTING

The "lid" of the toolbox will change with each new clinical rotation setting. Most lids will feel like a good fit. Some will be quite transparent—in other words, you will be able to see at a glance what tools you will need, what personal resources will be most relevant, and what you can expect to learn. Sometimes it will take a little more adjustment to get the new lid to fit. The following pointers will help you make those adjustments.

Clients/Patients

A new clinical rotation usually means a change in the type of clients with whom who will be working—different age groups, different levels of acuity, different health problems or diseases. To prepare for the new client/patient mix you may need to reorient yourself (e.g., from dealing with seniors to communicating with children). More fundamentally, the definition of client may be different. After two or three rotations in which clients have been acutely ill adults your thinking has been oriented to individuals. While you will have thought about their needs in the context of their families and community it can be quite different to go into a practicum where the client *is* the community. In this case, individuals become to the community what different body parts are to the individual. That takes some adjustment.

Lines of Communication

Finding out who's who and where they fit in formal and informal lines of communication should be a priority at the beginning of each clinical rotation. Early in your program this may involve only a few key people identified for you by your instructor (e.g., the nursing manager, the unit clerk or secretary, and the nursing staff with whom you will be working). Being able to address these people appropriately by the names they prefer, and knowing their job titles and roles is part of showing respect. Each time you have a question you should make an active decision as to whom it would be most appropriately addressed—the person most available is not necessarily the person most appropriate. It is usually *not* appropriate to go directly to the nursing manager with questions about patient care, location and use of equipment, and so on. Questions about assessments and clinical judgements are usually best discussed with your instructor and/or the staff nurse who is responsible for the clients/patients with whom you are working. If not resolvable at that level, the nursing manager or another health provider may then become involved. Questions about your own learning and curiosity may need to wait for your instructor. Most health-care providers enjoy doing a certain amount of informal teaching although their time to do so may be limited. How and when you ask is important.

As a student you are a guest in the agency. Sometimes you will be older than some of the staff, know one or two of them because of mutual interests, and so on. But remember that your role in this environment is that of a learner, not a colleague. It is better to err on the side of being reserved than to assume that because they laugh and joke with each other that it is okay for you to join right in. The secret is to be friendly

Notes

but not presumptuous of relationships. If, on the other hand, it is your tendency to be quiet and withdrawn, you may need to make an effort to be a little more outgoing and spontaneous, to not take your learning too seriously.

In clinical rotations later in your nursing program you will probably have more responsibility for communicating directly with a variety of health-care professionals, agency representatives, and others. A copy of the organizational structure can be very helpful in those situations. One of your learning objectives might be to analyze the formal and informal lines of communication as part of a program planning initiative.

Policies and Procedures

As a nursing student in a clinical rotation you are accountable to two sets of policies and procedures: those of your nursing program and those of the agency.

Dress Code.   Dress codes vary because of agency preferences, types of clients served, traditions, and values. For example, wearing your usual student name tag which identifies you by first and last name may violate policy in an emergency unit or a correctional institution. Such a regulation is for your personal protection. Other times regulations about what you may or may not wear have their origins in beliefs about what constitutes professionalism or the degree to which nurses should stand apart from or blend into the client population. Asking in advance as to what is appropriate can save you from later problems or embarrassment.

What You Can and Cannot Do.   There may be a core set of policies established by your nursing program affecting what you are allowed to do in clinical rotations. There may also be policies regarding what you can do as a student that have been established by the agency. For example, your nursing program may have policies as to what intravenous medications students in their final year are allowed to administer. You may have regularly administered a particular medication in a previous clinical rotation. If, however, the current practicum setting has a policy that only registered nurses certified for that medication can administer it, then you are bound by that policy—the lid of your toolbox has changed.

Remember that you are also guided in what you can and cannot do by the professional code of ethics. The International Council of Nurses Code of Ethics specifies that nurses must use judgement in relation to individual competence when accepting responsibilities (see Appendix A). Even if, by the policies of your nursing program and the agency, you are allowed to do something you must not do it unsupervised if you have not done it under supervision before or are not yet competent to do it alone.

Injuries and Exposures.   Nursing practice is not without its risks and you will want to know what procedures are to be followed should you be injured or exposed to infection, radiation, abuse, and so on. There will be a contract of some sort between your nursing program and the agency to provide for such possibilities. In instructor-led practica you can rely on your instructors to help you work through such a situation should it occur. In preceptored rotations, however, you and your preceptor will want to know what to do should you be injured at work. In this instance, minor injuries are actually more complicated than major ones. If you are seriously hurt you will usually be attended to by the agency until you can be transferred to an appropriate emergency department. However, in the event of a minor injury or an exposure such as a needlestick injury, you will want to know who is responsible to provide immediate treatment and follow-up.

Resources

Each time you start a clinical rotation in a new site you will want to find out what resources will be available to you. Where can you park your car? Are there special parking rates for nursing students? Is there a cafeteria? Are you eligible for the staff discount? Are lockers available? Ask about other resources such as access to the agency library. Sometimes even small agencies have a remarkable collection of resources specific to their focus (e.g., suicide prevention). Knowing about these resources can come in handy later, even for assignments in some of your more advanced theory courses.

ਟੇ SUMMARY

This chapter has been about getting your toolbox in order:

ਟੇ learning about learning as the foundation or bottom of your toolbox
— recognizing your learning preferences
— differentiating between learning-that and learning-how
— knowing the different stages of becoming competent in psychomotor skills
— thinking about questions for and from your clinical instructor

ਟੇ thinking about your personal resources as the sides of your toolbox
— feelings
— interests
— experiences
— capabilities

ਟੇ recognizing the practicum setting as the lid for your toolbox, something that changes with each rotation
— thinking about how the clients/patients will be similar or different to previous rotations
— getting to know the appropriate lines of communication
— finding out about policies and procedures
— locating resources

LEARNING TOOL 3.1

Learning How

LEARNING FOCUS: Values Exploration

This exercise will help you gain an understanding of the values you associate with "learning-how" to be a nurse. In particular, you will have a chance to put your feelings about your progress with psychomotor and other skills in perspective.

STUDENT ACTION

Think about your mental images of nurses in action, your expectations of yourself, and what you believe others expect of you.

1. Visualize a highly competent nurse working in your current practicum setting. Based on your image, complete the following chart, indicating the skill being performed and how the nurse performs the skill. For example:

What skills does the nurse perform?	How does the nurse perform the skill?
➤ listening to heart sounds	➤ calmly, without thinking
➤ managing IV therapy	
➤ conducting a family interview	

What skills does the nurse perform?   **How does the nurse perform the skill?**

2. Now visualize yourself in your current practicum context.

What skills do you perform?   **How do you perform the skill?**

3. Now that you have visualized an expert nurse and yourself in action, you can use one of the tools in this chapter, the Taxonomy of Psychomotor Behavior, to analyze your expectations. Make a list of the skills that you think you are expected to demonstrate in this practicum. For each skill listed, assess the level of proficiency that *you expect of yourself* and then assess the level of proficiency that *you think your instructor expects* of you for this skill.

For example,

Skills I think I am expected to perform in this practicum.	My expectation of myself.	My perception of instructor expectation.
❧ listening to heart sounds	❧ able to identify and name abnormal heart sounds, S_3, S_4, murmurs, clicks	❧ able to identify S_1 and S_2, tells what is normal and phase of cycle but not necessarily S_3, S_4, etc.

Skills I think I am expected to perform in this practicum.	My expectation of myself.	My perception of instructor expectation.

NOTES ON USE

Student Use.   This exercise can help you come to terms with what you expect of yourself and what you think others expect of you. A gap between how an experienced nurse does things and how you perform is to be expected. A gap between what you expect of yourself and what you think your instructor expects warrants further investigation. Discuss this gap with your instructor. Even if there is no gap, you may want to share your list with your instructor as a way of validating your expectations. Remember that your instructor has worked with many students at your level and thus will have a good sense of what is reasonable. However, this is your first time in this particular practicum so it is a little harder for you to know what is reasonable. On the other hand, you know yourself best and how well you have been able to do these and similar skills in the lab or in previous practica.

Instructor Use.   Skills checklists have been part of nursing education for many years but this exercise offers a new twist by helping students analyze their expectations. To take it a step further, you could have students use the Taxonomy of Psychomotor Behavior to set goals for the level of performance they will achieve by the end of the practicum. Or you might use this exercise as the basis for a one-to-one or group discussion of how expectations may differ and why that might happen. Students in preceptored settings may be particularly vulnerable to expecting that they need to reach the preceptor's level of skill, forgetting that the preceptor has years of experience.

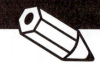

LEARNING TOOL 3.2

The Right Stuff

LEARNING FOCUS: Knowledge Building

This exercise extends your self-reflection on the interests, capabilities, and experiences you bring to clinical situations. In this exercise, you focus on qualities and capabilities you already have and use in your "everyday" life, which can hold you in good stead for any nursing situation.

STUDENT ACTION

1. For each capability, reflect upon past experiences (e.g., school, jobs, and leisure activities) that you associate with using the capability.
2. Identify your level of competence using the following scale:
   AA = above average
   A = average
   BA = below average
3. Describe at least one experience that validates your performance level assessment for all AA ratings (at a minimum).

For example:

Capability	Competence Level	Validating Experience
Be flexible	AA	Able to "go with the flow" when my boss keeps changing work procedures.

SELF-MANAGEMENT CAPABILITIES

Capability	Competence Level	Validating Experience
Be flexible		
Focus on task		
Show enthusiasm		
Take initiative		
Be self-disciplined		
Be resourceful		
Show a sense of humor		
Be thorough		
Demonstrate tact		
Perform under stress		
Be persistent		
Work as team member		

PROBLEM-SOLVING CAPABILITIES

Capability	Competence	Validating Experience
Analyze information		
Compile information		
Organize information		
Make decisions		
Develop hypotheses/hunches		
Monitor progress		
Able to troubleshoot		
Develop alternatives		

LEADERSHIP CAPABILITIES

Capability	Competence	Validating Experience
Coaching others		
Assessing situations		
Coordinating people/events		
Delegating to others		
Facilitating a group		
Handling complaints		
Motivating self/others		
Planning events		
Promoting a point of view		
Supervising others		
Working as a team		

CREATIVE CAPABILITIES

Capability	Competence	Validating Experience
Developing ideas		
Able to reframe ideas/situations		
Able to brainstorm		
Able to use things in several ways		

About which five of the capabilities you listed do you feel the most confident?

1.

2.

3.

LEARNING TOOL 3.2 continued

4.

5.

For which five capabilities would you like to improve your competence level?

1.

2.

3.

4.

5.

NOTES ON USE

Student Use.   These qualities and capacities form the sides of your learning toolbox. You can create a further visual record of these by decorating the sides of an actual box (e.g., shoe box) with the descriptive words that apply to you. You could type, print, or form the words from magazine or newspaper cutouts. This can be a fun project that reminds you of the strengths you bring to all clinical situations. We often overlook these qualities in ourselves and in others. Your clients/patients may also need to be reminded about the capabilities they bring to the challenging situations they face. This exercise will make a great addition to your practice portfolio (see Chapter 6).

Instructor Use.   This exercise focuses on the strengths students bring to clinical situations. You can use these strengths to increase students' motivation to learn through maintaining and enhancing their self-esteem. This might be a time to discuss how students will be called upon to use these capabilities to adapt to the varied clinical situations that are ahead. You can add categories of capabilities to those presented here and list skills or qualities that are related to each category. For example, more advanced students might explore "Making clinical judgements"; other categories include "Accessing information" (e.g., from human resources, libraries, research, Internet) or "Assertiveness."

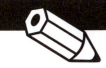

LEARNING TOOL 3.3

Thinking About Thinking About

LEARNING FOCUS: Critical Thinking Development

This exercise is about identifying personal preferences and strengths, as well as reflecting on the thinking process you use to identify these.

STUDENT ACTION

Answer the following questions about your preferences and strengths. Remember that there are no right or wrong answers. The purpose of this exercise is to increase your self-awareness and your ability to articulate your strengths and preferences. Many of the questions are phrased in either-or terms but you may feel that you have some of both—if so, write about that.

UNCOVERING TASK-RELATED PREFERENCES

1. How much variety do you need in your work?

2. Do you like to take over a messy situation and organize it *or* do you function better when a structure and organization are already in place?

3. Do you like to take complex situations, examine the parts, and show how the parts are interrelated *or* do you like to take an overview of many events and see how they fit together?

4. How do problems affect you?

5. What kind of problems get your creative or determined juices flowing (e.g., people problems, ideas, problems relating to things)?

6. Do you view problems as obstacles to be overcome, no matter what the cost, *or* do you tackle problems in off-beat or creative ways?

7. What are your work habits? Are you spontaneous, fairly disorganized, heedless of details *or* do you like to work in a methodical way?

8. What does creativity mean to you in the context of nursing?

UNCOVERING SELF-RELATED PREFERENCES

1. Do you prefer to work alone or in a group? How does your preference affect your performance in this clinical practicum?

2. How competitive are you? Rate yourself on a scale from one to ten.

3. Do you set high standards for yourself and compete with yourself?

4. Do you need competition to motivate yourself *or* are you more motivated by other things?

5. How do you handle yourself under stress—do you fall apart *or* do you thrive?

6. Do you tend to work to deadlines *or* do you like to plan and work far ahead?

7. How much feedback do you need about a project or assignment?

8. How much praise do you need to keep yourself going? How frequently and quickly do you need this positive feedback? What do you do if no praise is forthcoming?

9. Which events challenge you and which overwhelm you?

10. How important is status to you? Is it important for you to have ownership of an idea or project?

11. Do you enjoy persuading others about your ideas, concerns, or projects *or* do you prefer to act on other people's initiatives?

12. In making a decision, do you obtain large amounts of information or advice and ponder carefully all of the alternatives *or* do you follow your "inner sense" and make an instinctive decision? Do you decide quickly or ponder at length? Do you tend to decide things on your own *or* do you prefer to make shared decisions?

SUMMARIZING YOUR STRENGTHS

You have considered many aspects of yourself in the previous part of this exercise. Now it's time to examine the thinking processes you used in deciding what to choose out of the myriad possibilities.

1. What are your important strengths? Don't limit yourself to one area of your life (e.g., think of your educational life, social life, etc.).

2. What process did you use to determine your strengths? For example, did you start by naming various categories or roles? Perhaps your starting point was one area of your life and you went with whatever popped into your head.

3. How did you feel about looking at your strengths? Did your feelings change throughout the process?

4. What obstacles arose while you were identifying your strengths? How did you meet these challenges?

5. How could you use your strengths as strategies for effective learning? Don't limit yourself to professional strengths. Examine strengths from other areas of your life that could be helpful in your roles as a nursing student. For example, strengths with friends and family can be used in your relationships with classmates, expert nurses, and patients/clients.

NOTES ON USE

Student Use.   Here is more material for your practice portfolio. Knowing your own preferences will help you to understand why some assignments and situations are more or less difficult for you. Knowing your thinking processes and preferences will also help you to put differences between people within the context of preferred ways of learning, thinking, and doing. It is also important to know that you will not always be able to operate from your preferred way—which challenges you to grow! There are several theoretical perspectives from which to examine personality and learning style preferences (e.g., C. G. Jung's theory of psychological types and the

LEARNING TOOL 3.3 continued

Myers-Briggs Type Indicator [Myers, 1975]). You could add some of these ideas to the bottom of your learning toolbox for the learning process itself.

Instructor Use.   This exercise will give you an opportunity to examine your own preferences and relate them to your preferred way of instructing. Are you more comfortable using (1) a discussion method of teaching where you facilitate participation; (2) an information-giving method where you pass on your expert knowledge to students; (3) a coaching method where you facilitate active learning; or (4) a self-discovery method where learning is a co-evolving process. You can initiate a discussion about these and other methods of teaching and which of these methods are preferred by various students. The following quotation can help initiate a discussion on preferences:

At first the courses seemed a little too unstructured, but after giving it a chance, I think I like it better than just sitting and taking notes. My voice is important in the classroom and I know that when I'm inquiring about something or I want to make my position known, others are willing and interested to hear what I have to say.

NURSING STUDENT

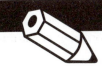

LEARNING TOOL 3.4

From a Strengths Perspective

LEARNING FOCUS: Application Enhancement

Now that you have some experience with identifying strengths, we would like you to apply this skill to a case. Notice the similarities and differences between identifying your own strengths and noticing the strengths of others.

STUDENT ACTION

As you read the case of Jason, remember you are looking for strengths. After reading, answer the questions.

> *Jason, a 32-year-old paraplegic who runs a small computer consulting business, has sought help from a mental health clinic because of recurrent depression. His most recent episode seems to have been precipitated by his girlfriend dumping him. Prior to his injury, he was an ambulance driver. His injury occurred five years ago in a work-related accident where the ambulance he was driving was hit by a driver who failed to stop at a stop sign. He had been an avid hiker, rock climber, and mountain bike enthusiast prior to his injury. In the last couple of years, he has become involved in a para-basketball league. He was working out at a local gym three times a week until about six weeks ago.*

1. What are Jason's strengths? Don't limit yourself to the health-related aspects of his life.

2. What was the process you used to determine his strengths?

3. How did you feel about looking at Jason's strengths? How did your feelings compare to looking at your own strengths?

4. What were the challenges that arose while you were identifying Jason's strengths?

5. How were these challenges similar or different from identifying your own strengths?

6. How might you use Jason's strengths in forming a care plan?

7. Is exploring strengths an ordinary focus of your assessment process with clients/patients? Why, why not?

8. Create a maxim that could serve as a reminder for focusing on strengths—your own and those of your patients/clients.

NOTES ON USE

Student Use.   Strengths can be quite "ordinary" capacities as you learned from previous exercises. Use this same framework for assessing the strengths of this client. Question 6 might best be worked on with a partner or in a small group; this way you can learn from each other's experiences.

Instructor Use.   Encourage students to draw examples of strengths that patients have from cases in their past or present clinical practicum. Some of these cases may become paradigm cases for the students. You might take this opportunity to discuss paradigm cases of your own and encourage students to be on the look-out for their own cases. Creating a maxim for this exercise can prompt student discussion and sharing of maxims.

LEARNING TOOL 3.5

Personalizing the Toolbox

JOURNAL FOCUS

You have spent a great deal of time and effort thinking and writing in the previous exercises for this chapter. This journal exercise is meant to tap into more "right-brain" aspects of your self. Have fun and be creative.

STUDENT ACTION

Draw the practicum toolbox as it was described at the beginning of this chapter. Draw the lid separately because you want to be able to fill the toolbox. From the previous exercises think about your personal resources that are holding up the toolbox and giving it form. Design stickers that represent some of your experiences, feelings, capabilities, and interests that could be put all over the sides of your *personalized* toolbox. Enjoy!

POSITIVE STATEMENTS ABOUT ME

Remember, at the end of each journal entry you are to draw out from your reflections and journal writing positive statements you can make about yourself. Make each statement an "I" statement.

NOTES ON USE

Student Use.   You can draw the toolbox or use the box you created for Learning Tool 3.2. Reviewing all the exercises from this chapter will help you draw out personal resources to form the stickers for this exercise. You might also ask friends, family, and classmates to describe your strengths and create stickers for your toolbox. Have them sign the stickers they create for you! You can use these reminders of your strengths from the eyes of others as reinforcements when the going gets tough.

Instructor Use.   You can make a display of the toolboxes created for this exercise. Have students share their feelings about creating and sharing their toolboxes with others. You can prepare a sticker or two for each student's toolbox in recognition of their capabilities as you see them. You can also invite students to create stickers for your own toolbox, showing how they perceive your strengths as an instructor. Suggest ways for the students to add to the top of the toolbox—the clinical rotation setting.

4

The Tools

JOURNAL THOUGHT

He taught me a lot about myself — as a nurse and a person. The experience with this patient increased my confidence and completely reinforced my love for becoming a nurse.

SECOND-YEAR NURSING STUDENT

This chapter is about strategies for success. A wide variety of tools may be useful but the ones we think are essential have to do with attitudes, learning plans, questioning, equipment, priorities, and self-care.

ATTITUDES, BELIEFS, AND EXPECTATIONS

Your attitudes about clinical practica are closely linked with your beliefs and expectations. Attitude has to do with how you approach something. Caring, openness, and curiosity are attitudes that contribute to success in nursing practice. Extremes of self-confidence or inferiority can detract from success.

The following scenario shows how the same set of personal resources (i.e., the four sides of your toolbox described in Chapter 3) may be expressed through different attitudes.

> *Jennifer, a 24-year-old nursing student, has worked as a lifeguard and competed in national swimming competitions. She has a passion for physiology, excitement, and travel. She knows she gets impatient easily and is dreading her practicum in a geriatric care center.*
>
> *On one hand, Jennifer may believe that there is not much to learn in working with elderly, chronically ill people in a nonacute setting. She may expect to be bored. She may have heard that the clinical instructor is gentle and caring, a strong advocate for the psychosocial needs of the elderly, but not strong in explaining the physiological aspects of aging and chronic illness. These beliefs and expectations may come across as an attitude of disinterest and even superiority.*

Notes

On the other hand, Jennifer may acknowledge her feelings but decide that she will try to be open about what there is to learn. She may believe that she will be more effective as a critical care nurse (which is what she wants to be) if she can learn to appreciate alternative perspectives. After all, elderly people do get admitted to intensive care units. She may be curious about the physiology of aging and decide to do some investigating on her own. She wonders if the instructor will be open to her doing a case study assignment with that focus. These beliefs and expectations come across as an attitude of curiosity and openness.

LEARNING PLANS

Often you will be expected to develop personal objectives and a learning plan for your clinical rotation. However, even if it is not a course requirement, developing a learning plan can be useful as a personal strategy for learning.

Identifying Your Learning Objectives

Start by identifying your own objectives for this practicum. Looking at the objectives in the course outline is a good place to start but then personalize them. Part of personalizing them is to consider your learning needs, interests, and career goals. Review your last clinical evaluation for areas to work on. One senior student identified her learning needs as:

- to become more confident in myself and my abilities;
- to be assertive in my decisions, actions, and ideas; and
- to develop increased sensitivity to ethical issues that affect nursing practice.

She went on to establish personal learning objectives that included: "To show evidence of increased confidence and assertiveness in dealing with clients and staff members through journaling." Another student identified a learning need related to improving comprehension and application of knowledge related to diagnostic testing. She described her learning objective as:

- To increase my knowledge of interpreting lab values and diagnostic results, how they relate to various illnesses, and the implications they have for nursing care.

Try to be as specific as you can. By wording objectives in such a way that they are measurable you will gain not only a sense of direction but also the ability to monitor your progress.

Organizing Your Learning Plan

The heart of your clinical learning plan is the creativity with which you identify and use resources and strategies to meet your objectives. Students often get stuck with a few routine strategies that have worked for them in the past. For example, you may believe that the best way to learn a new skill is to do it over and over. That may be a very good strategy but what happens if the number of opportunities is limited? Successful students realize that they can also learn in other ways such as carefully analyzing how someone else does a procedure, mentally rehearsing it at every step.

Refining Your Learning Plan

Build checkpoints into your learning plan. Some of those checkpoints are already scheduled, such as midterm and final evaluations. Other checkpoints can be of your own making. Reviewing and summarizing your journal entries at the end of the week is one type of checkpoint. Asking your instructor or preceptor for growth-oriented feedback specific to your personal objectives is another strategy. Keeping lists of clinical judgements made or counts of times you spoke up in postconference are more structured ways of monitoring progress.

The unpredictable nature of most clinical rotations makes it especially important to refine your learning plan as you go along. New learning needs and opportunities may emerge. On the other hand, you may find that some strategies are not feasible in a particular clinical setting. However, learning needs usually transcend more than one practicum so hang onto those strategies. They may be feasible in a later rotation. Noting changes to your learning plan in a different color of ink is one way to keep track of what is working and not working for this rotation.

❧ CRITICAL QUESTIONS

Questions help you to focus inquiry. In Chapter 1 we talked about five important words—who, when, where, how, and why—as essential traveling companions for the practicum process. In Chapter 3 we offered you a list of practical questions to use when starting a new clinical rotation. In this chapter we are thinking of reflective questions addressed to your instructor or others as tools to help your clinical learning, both "learning-how" and "learning-that."

Have you ever wondered what questions instructors wish you would ask? What questions other students ask their clinical instructors? Here are some ideas:

- ❧ What do you see as the most important thing to be learned from this situation?
- ❧ What do you see as the priorities for me in this situation?
- ❧ What problems should I anticipate?
- ❧ How might I have handled that situation differently?
- ❧ What would you have done?
- ❧ Why I am observing one thing (e.g., the way a procedure is done or an interview is handled, a patient's signs and symptoms, the type of lab tests ordered) but being told another (e.g., by the textbook; procedural manual; another nurse, the physician)? What is different about the two? Are they both right?
- ❧ Why do you think this situation is happening (e.g., vital signs are changing, adolescent is refusing a medication)? What other hypotheses could I consider?
- ❧ How can I make sense of this situation in the context of what we are learning about (e.g., conceptual frameworks, grief and loss, family processes)?

❧ EQUIPMENT

Having the equipment you need for clinical together and ready for use is a great stress reliever. The "How to Survive and Thrive in Clinical" set of tips that follows was written by a former student as part of her preparation for a new student orientation. The new students loved it and we thought you would find it useful too.

Notes

How to Survive and Thrive in Clinical

- Keep all the articles you routinely take to clinical in one bag set aside only for clinical. Once you have stocked it with the needed equipment, such as black pens, name tag, clinical shoes, stethoscope, etc., it is always ready provided you return the articles to the bag at the end of the day. This will prevent the stress of looking for all your stuff early in the morning or worse finding out that you left something needed at home.

- Buy a drug reference manual that comes in the form of recipe cards. This saves time because instead of writing out the drugs, you only have to look them up and take them out, as you need them. (Put the remainder in your clinical bag!) For more in-depth understanding of the drugs, consult your pharmacology text.

- To prepare for your patients, begin with your medical dictionary for a general description of their conditions. Next consult a handbook of care plans (available at the campus bookstore). It will summarize the typical care and things to be aware of when taking care of a patient with that condition. If you need a more in-depth understanding of a particular condition, consult your anatomy and physiology text or pathophysiology text. Finally, consult your nursing text for possible skills you may need to review and nursing care priorities.

- Remember that each clinical placement may be a potential employer in the future so try to be helpful to the nurses when you have a chance. Your willingness to assist them will be appreciated and create a positive working relationship.

- Develop a system of organizing your patient load. Some units have forms for the typical information you need to note, with spaces to record vitals and other assessment information, timelines for medications, etc. Get used to these and develop one that works for you. Then use it consistently.

- Practice your skills in the psychomotor skills lab. A typical complaint about the lab is that it is not like real life. This is valid, however, lab time can help you get the order of events down pat and therefore is helpful. You will be more confident with a real patient.

- Team up with another student and help each other do new things or solve problems together. Tasks seem easier when done together for the first time. (Subsequent attempts should be done on your own, if possible, to encourage independence.)

- Learn things right the first time. Make the most of tutorials. Study not just to pass a quiz but to remember the material later, or else you will have to start all over again.

- Go for it! Avoid taking "easy" patients out of fear. Doing things for the first time is always a little scary but in the end you will be better off for the experience. Remember that people will help you more when you are a student, so take advantage of their assistance.

- Remember that nurses who have been doing something for twenty years forget that even small tasks can be confusing to an inexperienced student. If they get annoyed or comment that you don't know something, gently remind them that you are new and that even the "easy" things are a challenge at first. Thank them for assisting you; help them with their busy day and they will be more inclined to help.

- Put your fear of making a mistake into perspective by asking your instructor to highlight some information that would be helpful at the beginning of each session. For example, "What are some of the mistakes that are likely to be made by a new student by accident?" "What are some of the guidelines for safe practice that you could highlight for this area?" This might flush out some of the particular concerns for each area.

🌢 Try to cut back the number of hours you put into your part-time jobs. It may be better to cut back your spending than to use up valuable spare time. It is very easy to burn out.

A very recent graduate

Uniforms and Such

At the start of your nursing program you may have received a list of uniform requirements. Here are a few more tips:

🌢 Get uniforms with big pockets, preferably not the slit type because things fall out.

🌢 Keep in mind that you will be:
— lifting . . . so look for ease of shoulder movement
— stooping over people . . . so check out what happens to the neckline when you bend over (no exposure please!)
— stretching . . . so avoid buttons because they have a tendency to gape at embarrassing moments
— Kneeling on beds and things . . . so look for ease of knee movement
— Perspiring . . . yes, nursing can be hard physical work so look for comfortable, cool fabrics
— Working nights . . . when a lab jacket is nice to slip over your uniform if the temperature drops
— Exposed to body fluids, dyes, etc. . . . so ease of washing and tolerance for hot water are musts.

🌢 Some practica will require clothing other than uniforms. Plan your wardrobe to include comfortable, professional-looking separates that will be suitable for home-care and community settings.

Accessories

Your name tag and a watch with a second hand are musts to have at all times. Nursing programs may have specific regulations about jewelry. Even if your program does not, keep the following points in mind:

🌢 Anything that dangles can be a source of injury to you. Young children and disoriented or aggressive adults have been known to grab and pull on loop earrings, necklaces, and such.

🌢 Rings (on fingers, in noses, and on other exposed body parts) can be a source of infection. Remember that you will be working at times with people whose immune systems are highly compromised. Any finger ring other than a plain band can potentially puncture a glove, exposing you and patients to the risk of infection.

🌢 Perfumes can trigger allergic reactions and contribute to nausea.

Stethoscopes and Things for Your Pockets

Buying your first stethoscope can be exciting. Get some advice and check out different ones. You do pay for quality. A really cheap one, especially if it has long extensions, can make auscultation skills harder than ever. On the other hand, stethoscopes do get lost and stolen so investing in a top-of-the-line model in your first year might not be wise either.

If you are preparing for your first practicum you might be wondering what you will be carrying in those big pockets! A pen (or two) and a notebook are musts. Sometimes agencies require that charting be done in a certain color of ink because of the need for copying or use of color-codes for different types of information. A penlight is useful especially if your practicum is in a critical care, emergency, or recovery room environment, or otherwise involves patients with neurological problems. Be sure you have fresh batteries. Bandage scissors are especially handy for 101 uses other than cutting bandages (which you will rarely have to do). Drug cards are a must. Cards are now available for both assessment and diagnostic procedures, or you may want to make up your own.

A pocket-sized notebook with replaceable pages is particularly handy because you may want to discard some notes at the end of a shift, while you may want to keep other information through several practica. The information you can carry in your notebook is next best to what you can carry in your head because it is with you at all times. Your notebook is a good place for:

- notes on organizing your patient load for the day;

- things you must remember to chart;

- microsummaries about common conditions;

- key points on things you mix up frequently (e.g., differences in symptoms between insulin reaction and diabetic coma, decerebrate versus decorticate posturing);

- formulas for calculating divided doses;

- common drug incompatibilities;

- assessment frameworks (e.g., the ABCs of emergencies); and

- sayings, maxims, or verses that are a quick source of strength to you.

PRIORITY SETTING

One of the most important tools for success is allowing yourself enough time to do well in your clinical practica. Jobs, family needs, and social life can complicate the clinical rotation part of your nursing education even more than other course work. You have juggled your studying with other areas of life in the past. By now you will have learned that cramming the night before the exam or starting a term paper the day before it is due generally does not work too well at this level. Though you might have gotten away with that approach earlier in your education, clinical practica raise other priority-setting issues.

It takes time to prepare for each practicum day and time to reflect afterwards. It is not just a matter of looking good in front of the instructor. Not knowing the action, side effects, contraindications, and maximum safe dosage of a medication could have serious consequences for a patient. You cannot afford to risk being inadequately prepared!

Scheduling clinical rotation hours is often not within your control but may conflict with a part-time job, day-care availability, and family expectations. You have chosen a nursing career and now need to arrange the other parts of your life to support that decision. That does not mean your family should be any less of a priority, but your children's swimming lessons may need to temporarily drop in importance. Likewise, you may need to negotiate adjustments with your employer, take a leave of absence, and/or seek alternative financial support. Many students feel they must work or are in situations that limit their choices. If you are not sure how to deal with your personal situation, talk it over with your instructors. They can probably direct you to other resource people in your educational institution if necessary. It also helps your instructors to understand some of your constraints. Occasionally, a modification can be made to your clinical rotation but it is not wise to count on that possibility.

ࢢ SELF-CARE

The preservation of health is a duty. Few seem conscious that there is such a thing as physical morality.

Herbert Spencer

Sleep

Getting adequate sleep is an important tool. Sleep helps with memory, concentration, energy, attitude, patience, problem solving, general health, and enjoyment of your clinical experiences. On the other hand, clinical rotations may disrupt your usual circadian rhythms. You may have to get up earlier or even work shifts. So, read on.

Sleep Hygiene.   Though a strange term to describe healthy sleep habits, good sleep hygiene has three fundamental principles:

ࢢ Maintain as regular a schedule as possible—that means not sleeping in for hours on the weekend to catch up because of the all-nighter you pulled to finish that last term paper.

ࢢ Make healthy choices about the amount and timing of stimulants—that means
  — chemicals such as coffee and chocolate because they may keep you awake;
  — exercise because, though it generally helps sleep, if done too close to bedtime it increases core temperature (sleep comes easiest when core temperature decreases);
  — working right up to bedtime with no wind-down period; and
  — worrying about things (yes you can schedule worry time but don't do it in the middle of the night).

ࢢ Make time for relaxation and getting enough sleep—that means giving your own needs some priority (people who enter the helping professions are notorious for feeling that other people's needs are more important than their own).

Adjusting to Shift Work.   Shift work often involves having to work when you should be sleeping and having to sleep when your body expects you to be awake. There are two sleep-related problems associated with shift work: difficulty sleeping during the day and difficulty staying alert at night. "Night people" generally adjust to shift work more easily than "morning people." Make child-care arrangements as though you were away at work or school. Often students will try to manage children and other responsibilities by napping while the children are away at school, being available for phone calls, or even catching up on errands at the expense of trying to sleep. After an evening shift, a wind-down period is especially important because those shifts are often busy right up to the time you report off. Go to sleep when you feel sleepy. After a night shift try to avoid being exposed to a lot of daylight; before going to sleep for example, you may choose to wear sunglasses on your way home and pull the blinds as soon as you get there. To encourage sleep during the day, darken your room as much as you can, disconnect the phone, and go to bed with an expectation that you will get a good sleep. A nap later in the day is advisable if you sleep for a few hours and then cannot get back to sleep.

Staying alert throughout the night can be a challenge. In industrial settings, it has been shown that the brighter the workplace the more alert workers are likely to be. However, the settings in which nurses work nights need to provide an environment that is supportive to sleep for patients. Bright lights in charting areas, medication rooms, and such can be helpful so long as they do not shine into patient areas. Keep active as much as you can. In some places nursing staff are allowed to take naps on their breaks. The effectiveness of this practice in restoring alertness is controversial. It may temporarily improve alertness or it may contribute to what is called sleep inertia, the sense of being unable to get going again at all. Sleep inertia is especially problematic in on-call situations where you may have to react immediately.

Attention to what and when you eat is also important as part of adjusting to shift-work. Small frequent meals may be helpful but avoid snacking as a substitute for eating well-balanced meals. Choose foods high in protein and carbohydrates; avoid fried foods and hard-to-digest meals.

Exercise

Nursing students tend to polarize in the attention they give exercise as part of self-care. Many students work out regularly, sometimes pushing themselves too hard. Other students feel they have no time or energy left for exercise. If you are part of the latter group, it is time to reevaluate your priorities. Like sleep, exercise can improve concentration, energy, attitude, patience, problem solving, general health, and enjoyment of life. Regular exercise also improves stamina, which is important given the physical and emotional demands inherent in the nursing profession.

Nutrition

You have learned about the importance of good nutrition as part of your nursing program. You probably have good intentions but may have found that barriers get in the way. Your hectic schedule may mean that you are often away from home at what would be your usual meal times. You may feel that you don't have time to cook or even to shop. These are matters of priority setting—of valuing yourself and your health enough to make some adjustments. However, some of you may not be able to afford adequate food. Students in this situation are often embarrassed and go without even though there are resources available. If you are in this situation talk to your instructors; they will help you.

Relaxation

A major part of self-care is providing for relaxation and stress reduction. Given the intensity of most clinical rotations, the pressures to keep up with your other courses, and everything else going on in your life, time for relaxation may get crowded out. Things that used to be relaxing may now seem like just one more thing to do. Maybe you really like classical music but have been noticing that even when you do take in a performance you end up thinking about the case study you haven't finished instead of immersing yourself in the music. Working through the learning tools at the end of this chapter may help you get reconnected with meeting your relaxation needs.

ASSERTIVENESS AND PERSONAL PROTECTION

Another tool for your clinical rotation toolbox has to do with your resources for assertiveness and personal protection.

Assertiveness

Assertiveness is such an important skill for nurses that many programs have included assertiveness training in their curricula. The ability to be assertive, rather than passive or aggressive, is a useful skill for anyone. What makes assertiveness so important in the helping professions is its link to being an effective advocate for the clients with whom we work. How assertive are you? Can you intervene in such a way that your client's needs are met? Situations that call for assertiveness will emerge in any clinical context. Consider this scenario:

> *Mrs. Humphrey had been on antidepressant medication for the past four months. She was admitted to hospital four days ago with a bowel obstruction. Now that she is recovering from surgery she is asking about her antidepressant medication. She is concerned that it has not been restarted. You tried to ask the surgical resident when she made rounds this morning but she brushed the concern off as unimportant saying Mrs. Humphrey can worry about that when she gets home.*

What would you do next?

Safety

Protecting yourself is a legitimate concern as you engage in clinical rotations. Some ways to protect yourself, such as universal precautions, may be thoroughly taught in your program. Nevertheless, it is up to you to use that knowledge and to consistently follow the recommended procedures. Other issues of personal protection, such as how to handle aggressive behavior, may be dealt with in class but still leave you feeling uncomfortable. Talk through these concerns with your instructor. Watch how your instructor or preceptor handles such situations in the clinical area. Suggest personal protection as a topic for postconference.

Occasionally a student may feel unsafe in other ways. You may find that you are taking a lot of emotional issues home from your clinical experiences. You will encounter many emotionally charged situations. Learning to debrief with someone appropriate (your instructor, a peer, a counselor) will help you to contain the emotional intensity. You may also need to seek out other strategies for reestablishing your emotional boundaries.

❧ SUMMARY

In this chapter we have considered different types of tools for building success in clinical rotations. The tools we have talked about are:

- ❧ checking out attitudes, beliefs, and expectations;
- ❧ developing a personalized learning plan;
- ❧ asking critical questions;
- ❧ having the right equipment in the right place at the right time;
- ❧ setting priorities;
- ❧ self-care; and
- ❧ assertiveness and personal protection.

Success in clinical rotations is an integral part of your entire nursing program so we conclude this chapter with more words of wisdom from a former student.

Notes

How to Survive and Thrive in General

- Get enough sleep! This is not an option! Nursing is challenging enough; without sleep, getting through the day is not only torture but is unsafe practice as well.

- Foster friendships with other students and keep those friendships healthy. Be the kind of friend you want to have.

- Participate in student functions. Students who excel often are the ones that have a rounded participation in the program. The more you get involved the more people you meet and are able to network with. Generally, nurses are kind, approachable people. Resist the temptation to watch movies or TV on the weekend rather than getting out. It's worth the effort. Remember you are responsible for making student functions fun. Get your friends to come, plan to have fun and you won't be disappointed.

- It is inevitable that you will have an occasional bad day. Sit back, take some time to reflect, regroup, and to decide how you will handle things next time. Or just cry. A good cry is great for giving you perspective. Discuss your concerns with your nursing instructor, etc. They can be of great help—don't "save face" and/or marks and miss out on getting the help you need. Nursing is a very demanding profession and it requires us to use all of ourselves. Sometimes the emotional drain is too much and you need to step back and take some deep breaths. It doesn't mean that you are a horrible nurse when you have a bad day. Just prove yourself the next day. Things will get better if you make them better.

- Be proud of the contribution you make to the care of patients. As a nursing student you may take more time than an experienced nurse but you have something unique to offer. Nursing students often have the time and enthusiasm to do the little TLC things that a nurse with a full load does not have time for—so it evens out!

Good luck. Going to nursing school will facilitate an enormous amount of personal growth and will connect you to many close friends. You are in for a very interesting and challenging four years.

A very recent graduate

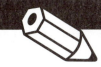

LEARNING TOOL 4.1

Checking Out Expectations

LEARNING FOCUS: Values Exploration

At the beginning of this chapter, we gave you two versions of Jennifer's attitudes and expectations going into a clinical rotation that were not related to her "real" interests. This exercise will help you personalize the difference attitudes and expectations can have on what you bring to a clinical experience, how patients/clients may perceive you, and what you take from the experience.

STUDENT ACTION

Think about your major area of interest in nursing. Now, think about your preferred context for practicing your interest area. Remember that we are still talking about preferences and ideals here!

1. Write down your major area of interest in nursing and your preferred context in which you would like to practice.

2. What personal experiences and qualities would you bring to your interest area of nursing that make you particularly suitable for this type of nursing?

3. What qualities would you like to portray in your preferred practice setting?

4. Consider an area of nursing that would seemingly be unrelated to your interest area—as geriatric nursing in a nursing home setting is for Jennifer. Write it down here.

5. What would your immediate reaction be to an assignment to this very clinical practicum? Express your thoughts and feelings. Remember, honesty is the best policy.

6. How might you come across to patients/clients and staff members in that setting, if you do not modify your thinking?

7. How could you change your immediate reaction to more closely resemble the qualities you would like to portray in your preferred practicum?

NOTES ON USE

Student Use.   It is essential that you not let your inner censor filter your immediate reactions in situations, such as being assigned to a clinical rotation that seems far removed from your ideal. Allowing those negative thoughts to emerge into consciousness is an important part of giving yourself the gift of growing. The strategies you develop for changing your attitude and expectations may seem like a stretch, but stretching exercises are a great way of warming up for strength and endurance exercises. Although this exercise generates highly personal reflections, sharing your thoughts and strategies with someone else will enrich your learning. Remember that you have much to give and much to learn.

Instructor Use.   Self-disclosure on your part may be appropriate before asking students to share these rather personal thoughts in small groups. Draw on your own experiences and those of former students. Teach by modeling the benefits of self-disclosure. This will help to set the stage for students to come to you, or others in authority, when they need to share about mistakes made in the practicum setting. It also will affirm the importance of self-disclosure for addressing mistakes. There are two issues to be conscious of before initiating such a discussion. First, the discussion may raise discomforting emotions for students, so be aware that some may need help putting themselves back together before leaving the classroom. Second, talk about the issue of confidentiality before beginning any discussion in which students are asked to reveal parts of themselves. Addressing these issues will inform students about your respect and support in disclosing personal information.

LEARNING TOOL 4.2

Your Early Warning System

LEARNING FOCUS: Knowledge Building

Stress is a natural part of life. It can push or pull us into changing our lives. However, there are times when stress seems to run our lives, which can lead to illness or most certainly sap our energies. This exercise is designed to assist you in exploring many facets of stress and stress management.

STUDENT ACTION

1. Add to the following lists of signs and symptoms of stress.

Physical	Emotional	Cognitive	Behavioral
Leg movements	Mood swings	Foggy thinking	Decreased exercise
Nail biting	Anxiety	Mental blocks	Increased smoking
Tight shoulders	Anger	Disorganized	Increased caffeine use
Dry mouth	Withdrawal	Increased errors	Difficulty sitting still
Heart pounding	Apathy	Daydreaming	Easily startled

2. What are your typical signs of stress? Do you have an "early warning system" that alerts you to approaching overload? What are the early signs for you?

3. Here are some visualizations that may help decrease your anxiety level when you first clue into the rising tide of anxiety. They require you to use your imagination to change your feelings. You can use them while riding the bus or while taking a bathroom break.

   🙌 Sit in a comfortable position.

   🙌 Close your eyes.

❧ Breathe out and in three times—do this slowly and consciously. Controlled breathing helps you control your anxiety level. Start to let out long, slow exhalations through your mouth, and take in normal, not exaggerated inhalations through your nose. Do not take big, deep inhalations as this will increase your anxiety and may make you feel faint.

❧ Picture yourself _____
   — feeding powerful giants
   — making friends with hostile beings
   — calling forth hidden inhabitants of a cavern
   — facing ghosts in an old castle
   — seeing how, in order to fulfill yourself, you have to struggle with the tide
   — looking into clear, quiet, calm water and seeing what you wish to see

or

❧ Visualize yourself entering a desert carrying a backpack. As you walk, you notice darkness looming ahead of you. You know this means that a sandstorm of anxiety is coming toward you. As it approaches, picture yourself removing a folded tent from your backpack. Unfold it and set it up, driving the four pegs into place, raising the tent, then going in through the flap and closing it behind you. Sit peacefully in your tent as you hear the sand blowing around and over the tent. Know that when you hear the sandstorm pass completely, your anxiety has passed.

❧ Open your eyes.

4. What was it like for you as you visualized the anxiety passing?

5. In what situations could you use this or a similar exercise with patients/clients?

NOTES ON USE

Student Use.   These are techniques that you can teach clients and patients as well as family and friends. You may want to write some suggestions on a card to carry with you. Have friends and colleagues know your stress responses and give them permission to make you aware that "you're doing it again" (e.g., twirling your hair or jiggling your left leg)! Congratulate yourself on handling even mildly stressing events or situations. Share with others and ask them to congratulate you on the way you are learning and growing. We all need positive strokes. Ask for them if they are not coming your way.

Instructor Use.   Stress management must be part of your life, so share a few of your stress-busting gems. Make stress management practical by drawing upon real-life cases or situations in the practicum. Role playing and behavioral rehearsal may be useful teaching strategies for small group work in the area of stress management. Extending this exercise to what and how students can share with clients in this practicum about simple stress management techniques is also useful. In turn, this may provoke a discussion on assessing patient stress as part of care planning.

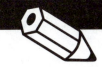

LEARNING TOOL 4.3

Meltdown—Stress Out of Control!

LEARNING FOCUS: Critical Thinking Development

Preventing burnout means handling stress in creative and resourceful ways. Avoiding all stress provoking situations is not possible, however, you can develop strategies that will help you manage stress more effectively. Juggling the demands of course work, clinical, family responsibilities, and a social life can present you with a monumental task. Establishing personal and professional goals will help you to manage time of stress better.

STUDENT ACTION

Here you are asked to articulate goals, time frame, strategies, and trade-offs for each of the major "demand" areas in your life just now: course work, clinical, family, and social life.

COURSE WORK

Goals: (e.g., "Obtain a minimum grade of B in each course.")

Time Frame: (e.g., 6 hrs/week class time; 15 hrs/week study time)

Strategies: (e.g., "Use the psychomotor lab more frequently. Set aside Saturdays from 9:00 AM to 3:00 PM to work on written assignments for the next week.")

Trade-Offs: (e.g., "I will trade off aiming for an A grade in order to spend more time on clinical practicum issues.")

LEARNING TOOL 4.3 continued

CLINICAL ROTATION

Goals: (e.g., "Come prepared for each clinical day.")

Time Frame: (e.g., "Spend at least 1 hour the night before clinical preparing for the next day.")

Strategies: (e.g., "Make notes during shift report.")

Trade-Offs: (e.g., Trade-off going out the night before a new practicum for some peace of mind.)

FAMILY

Goals: (e.g., "Stay connected to family yet remain independent.")

Time Frame: (e.g., 3 to 5 hrs/week; holidays)

Strategies: (e.g., "See parents once a week and call several times.")

Trade-Offs: (e.g., During exams, call parents but don't see them.)

SOCIAL LIFE

Goals: (e.g., Stay connected with friends who are not in nursing.)

Time Frame: (e.g., Friday nights are for me.)

Strategies: (e.g., Pre-arrange meeting up with friends on Friday.)

Trade-Offs: (e.g., During exam times, limit myself to *just* Friday nights for socializing.)

1. Time management is a key to stress management. At certain times the demands of course work and clinical practicum will accelerate. Under what circumstances would you expect course or clinical practicum work to take top priority in terms of time? How would you plan for these times of high stress and competing demands?

2. Have outlets to relieve your stress. How do you usually cope in times of stress (e.g., eat, sleep, or exercise)? How can you consciously incorporate these into your goals and strategies as defined in the early part of this exercise?

3. Throughout your student nursing experience, you may occasionally want to "throw in the towel." How will you cope with this sentiment? What counter-thoughts could you use to put things in a better perspective? Do you have a maxim or two that might help you to refocus, such as "this too will pass"? Keep in mind that what we tell ourselves about our experience can lessen the impact of stressful situations.

LEARNING TOOL 4.3 continued

NOTES ON USE

Student Use.   This exercise is based on stress and cognitive-behavioral theory. Its process is very similar to the process of writing learning objectives or personalizing learning objectives set out by your program. Both processes require you to articulate the ways in which you intend to accomplish your goals or the objectives of your program. Trade-offs are an important part of these considerations and related to priority setting described in the early part of the chapter. Just as you can't be all things to all patients, you can't do everything in the way or the proportion you would prefer. More often than not, you will have to make hard choices. Your values and expectations will guide you in these choices.

Instructor Use.   You can help students break things down into small steps by making to-do lists and then prioritizing items. Remind students that *doing* can be a great stress reliever. This might be an excellent time to highlight learning styles and their relationship to stress and stress reduction. One important issue to discuss with students is that when we are under pressure we tend to feel much more comfortable with our preferred ways than with ways that are not within our preferred spectrum. Students may find themselves more critical at these times of other ways and this can be normalized for them. You can link this exercise's goal writing to their learning agreements or expectations upon which they will be evaluated.

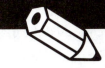

LEARNING TOOL 4.4

Assert Yourself!

LEARNING FOCUS: Application Enhancement

This exercise centers on assertiveness and personal protection. Assertiveness provides a format for you to request what you want and need. Just like yourself, clients may need to be encouraged to be assertive.

STUDENT ACTION

The following statements are about being assertive. After each statement, give examples as indicated.

1. Speak up while your want is current—don't wait until it is too late! Give an example of when you have done this in the past and an example of when this is difficult for you to do (e.g., when talking to my mother-in-law).

2. Be specific about behavior that you feel/think infringes on your rights. Avoid over-generalizing. Give an example of a recent experience where your rights have been infringed.

3. Assertiveness is about being brief and to the point. Write a plan for being brief and to the point about an academic or clinical situation in which you have or might need to be assertive with someone in authority.

4. Stay with the present situation—don't bring up the past. Write an example of when someone used the past instead of staying in the present situation with you.

5. Never apologize for asserting your rights—you have the right to ask for what you want, even though you may not always get it. Develop a list of nursing student rights, then a list of client rights.

6. Tell others how their behavior affects you—be sure to share how you feel. The communication process can be helped by using the following formula: (1) describe the specific behavior; (2) describe how you interpreted that behavior; and then, (3) describe how your interpretation made you feel. For example: "(1) When you left the room as soon as I came in, (2) I thought that you must still be angry with me, (3) so I was really upset." Now you write an example.

7. Assertiveness is expressed not only by what you say but also by your body movements, your eyes, your facial expressions, and especially your tone of voice. Describe how each of these nonverbal expressions would look like for you when you are being assertive rather than passive.

8. We have all received socialization messages growing up as well as in professional contexts. Some of the following may be familiar messages to you. These socialization messages can affect your ability to act assertively. For each, write how this message would help and/or hinder your being assertive.

    ❧ Be understanding and overlook trivial irritations. Don't be a complainer.

    ❧ Help other people. Don't be demanding.

    ❧ Be sensitive to other people's feelings. Protect others from the hard feelings.

    ❧ Think of others first; give to others even if you're hurting. Don't be selfish.

▸ Be modest and humble. Don't act superior to other people.

NOTES ON USE

Student Use.   Asserting yourself with some people, especially those in authority, can be difficult. Behavior rehearsal can give you the experience to face the real thing! Practice with classmates or friends. Monitor your self-talk in situations where you hesitate to be assertive, which can give you insight into what is holding you back. Perhaps it will be some socialization message from your past that may no longer be serving you well.

Instructor Use.   This is a good time to remind students that assertive behavior can have both positive and negative outcomes. Ask students to work in pairs or small groups to come up with examples of positive and negative outcomes they have experienced while being assertive. Students can also present scenarios to the class illustrating these examples, with others giving feedback on how the situations were handled. In giving feedback, students should be encouraged to use guidelines that promote more open communication: (1) describe the action in specific behavioral terms; (2) explain the results of that behavior; and (3), if appropriate, offer suggestions for improvement. Remind students that feedback can also be both positive and negative. If the feedback is positive, give the receiver time to revel in it.

Client rights and patient assertiveness are important issues to discuss with students. Students can be asked to come up with possible socialization messages that might be at play in client-nurse situations. You might also discuss the personal, cultural, and institutional barriers faced by clients/patients and how to assess these.

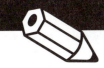

LEARNING TOOL 4.5

The First Is the Hardest

JOURNAL FOCUS

Here is a journal entry for you to reflect upon. Perhaps it will touch off a memory of your first experience with someone dying—either in clinical or in your personal experience.

This journal entry will probably be the hardest one for me to write; I feel like crying outright. I am definitely crying inside, yet part of me is "happy"! I was prepared to write about how confident, prepared, and good I felt about the whole week. Upon opening the Sunday paper and turning to the obituaries, there was my patient's name in front of me. I couldn't believe it! It was really a shock as I hadn't expected it so soon and was looking forward to being with him this week. I have many feelings about his passing as death has been on my mind lately (not that it scares me any longer).

This is the first patient I have ever lost. I guess the first is always the hardest. I certainly won't forget the whole experience. I cut out his obituary and plan to save it.

I wonder what he was like before the stroke — could he hear me, did he feel me squeezing his hand? I wish I could have been there.

He taught me a lot about myself — as a nurse and a person. The experience with this patient increased my confidence and completely reinforced my love for being a nurse. I am unsure how I feel. I may feel totally different tomorrow — I'm going to sleep on it.

SECOND-YEAR NURSING STUDENT

JOURNAL WRITING

Montgomery (1993) suggests that ". . . the very nature of caring implies that caregivers open themselves up to the experience of vulnerability. . . . [Caregivers feel] the personal loss and emotional pain that goes with grief; however, in most cases, the grief is also felt as a personally enriching experience" (pp. 106–107).

1. Write about a grief experience from your personal or clinical experience.

2. Was this, or did this become, a personally enriching experience? Why or why not? In what ways did the experience enrich you?

3. How did you get from grief to personal enrichment? What was your process? Was there more to it than the passage of time?

4. Were there other resources or other ways that might have made processing the grief experience more fruitful? What difference do you think these would have made?

POSITIVE STATEMENTS ABOUT ME

Remember, at the end of each journal entry you are to draw out from your reflections and journal writing positive statements you can make about yourself. Make each statement an "I" statement.

NOTES ON USE

Student Use.   Writing about emotionally intense experiences can take a lot of energy. Give yourself some recovery time after this journal writing. Do some self-care, whether alone or with others. Writing down such experiences helps to externalize the feelings and can give you a bit of distance to put things in perspective. Grief and loss theory can inform your experience as well as grief experiences of your clients.

Instructor Use.   Watch for and reinforce the unique ways in which students approach such an exercise. You might be able to help them see such differences from a preferred way of learning perspective. This helps to reinforce that it's okay to do some things in a different way. Having students share experiences in small- and large-group settings can be helpful in allowing them to review the experience with less emotional intensity. You might suggest that they ask other experienced nurses about their death and dying memories.

PART THREE

Tools of the
Profession

5

Learning in a Supervised Context

JOURNAL THOUGHT

This week was great. I had a nice patient and a great primary nurse to work with. She took the time to explain things to me and let me do things that she didn't have to (i.e., take out an IV). She let me listen to the lungs of a patient who had fluid in them and the bowel sounds of another. They were not my patients, but she really wanted me to have the experience. . . . One of the last things she said to me before I left was that she hoped I would love nursing as much as she does.

NURSING STUDENT, IN THE INITIAL PRACTICUM

Your practica are some of the best parts of learning professional nursing practice. You will learn more about practice and working with people from your instructors and other experienced nurses than from most books you will consult. Your instructors are not only *experienced* nurses, they are *expert* nurses in the thinking and doing elements of nursing practice. The relationships you develop with your instructors are instrumental to the process of learning to become a nurse. Practica provide a supervised learning context that assists you integrating nursing practice, your thinking skills, and content knowledge. Your instructors will consistently challenge your ability in areas of assessing, planning, implementing, and evaluating as you perform your work. They examine your daily activities and use these opportunities to provide teaching moments. Learning in a supervised context is a primary source of your evolving expertise—the context that assists nursing students to access multiple sources of knowledge and attain understanding about the caring process.

WHAT TO LEARN, HOW TO LEARN?

The process by which one moves from novice to expert nurse is related to accessing the knowledge that instructors and experienced nurses have about the practice of nursing. Where do you start? What do you learn and what is to be learned? Naturally, you will be expanding your content knowledge, but learning is also about reflecting on realities through examples of planned and unplanned practices. While this is a highly individualized process, it involves drawing on your senses—hearing, thinking, feeling, and doing— by capturing your experiences through writing, describing, reading, and reacting.

One of the first steps is focus on your learning or thinking style. The process is about building on your thinking style and discovering your patterns of acquiring knowledge. Your learning style may or may not be the same as another student. This is why different students often approach tasks in different but equally effective ways. It is why you prefer certain types of assignments—presentations versus essays, case studies versus critical analysis. You should not view differences as right or wrong. Instead, you need to identify your thinking style and recognize the practicum teaching style so that you can effectively accommodate your way of understanding. This is important because you will learn from your instructor that there are different ways of understanding and thinking about nursing situations and the material you are learning.

Different Ways of Understanding

Learning style refers to how you focus your attention, gather information, and make decisions. It is helpful in promoting understanding of you and others. Most students have a preferred approach to learning. If you do not know what your preferred approach is, there are a number of well-known tools available for identifying learning styles (Sarasin, 1998). Essentially the general characteristics between the various tools describe learners as having preferred approaches to auditory, visual, and tactile techniques to learning. You may find it helpful to access one of these tools to verify what you think is your preferred approach to learning. Your instructor may be able to suggest a preferred tool used in your nursing program. If not, consider your own abilities and preferences. One common tool to identifying your approach is the Kolb (The Teaching Professor) Inventory—diverger, converger, accommodator, and assimilator.

Diverger.   Students with this preferred approach to learning perceive information from concrete experiences. Divergers need to express their feelings and want to see things from different perspectives. Discussions and interactions with instructors and others are important to understanding. If you are a diverger, your strength will be generating ideas. It is recommended that you use the following tools for learning:

- Take advantage of opportunities to borrow equipment for psychomotor skills and try it out in different situations.
- Use free forms of writing to record ideas.
- Ask yourself "why" questions as you search to understand the importance of a nursing task or concept.
- Review materials, cases, and ideas with peers.
- Share personal reactions and opinions with your instructors and peers to clarify issues about clinical situations and the nursing process.

Converger.   If your preferred approach to learning is as a converger, you will like to learn by doing and may find it difficult when the situation is ambiguous and there is no one "right" response. You like to try things first. Practicality and usefulness are also key issues to your understanding. Your strengths are that you make decisions quickly, prefer one right answer, and are able to detect the essential aspects of a case or piece of practice. You also prefer to work alone as you learn. It is recommended that you use the following tools for learning:

- Volunteer to do skills in the lab and in the practice context.
- Write problem-solving protocols in your notebook.
- Review notes to see patterns and understand the method or approach to nursing practice.
- Write or record ways to improve skills and clinical problem solving in your day-to-day practice.
- Access case studies or simulations to prepare for practice.

Accommodator.   If this is your preferred learning approach you like to learn and think through self-discovery. Given a situation or problem, you will do best when you can create something new with it. You learn from mistakes and are identified as a problem solver or risk taker. Students with this learning style accommodate or adapt what they have learned to other situations, often improving on it. As an accommodator, you will use your instructor as a resource because you prefer less direct guidance. You are also a good teacher. It is recommended that you use the following tools for learning:

- Take advantage of problem-solving opportunities in handling equipment and in modifying procedures for different situations (e.g. how would it be different to take blood pressure for the elderly versus a toddler?).
- Explain or discuss how you solved a problem to other students.
- Write an explanation for solving a dilemma in nursing practice or in a client situation.
- Write a one-page description of innovative ways to intervene in a particular area of nursing practice.
- Approach learning in an open-ended manner.

Assimilator.   If you have the assimilator style of learning you will prefer first to reflect and observe. Gaining a conceptual understanding, then learning from experts through reading, listening, and lectures are ways you approach your thinking. You prefer well-organized situations, details, and good directions because you like to analyze pieces of information. It is recommended that you use the following tools for learning:

- Take advantage of teaching videos, procedure manuals, and other learning resources to prepare for doing psychomotor skills.
- Employ mapping techniques and graphic tools to help your learning.
- Use summaries and highlights to build on your strengths.
- Write after thinking and reflecting.
- In lab, find an accommodator as a partner; you will be particularly helpful first as an observer to give feedback.

    These are only some suggestions to aid your learning and development. You may likely find that you use a combination of thinking styles, with one style more dominant than the others. You will then need to draw on various methods to enhance learning. You are already aware of the ways or habits you have in your approach to learning.

Source of Expertise

Now that you have an understanding and awareness of your learning style, your instructor can support what you do best and understand your strengths and skills, as

Notes

well as your needs, wants, and knowledge gaps. Both you and your practicum instructor are sources of expertise. Building on your knowledge strengths will help you advance your critical thinking skills. An effective practicum instructor will try to accommodate to how you learn. From your peers, many of whom will have different learning styles, you will come to appreciate alternative ways of learning. Supervision from an experienced nurse—your instructor—is a key to the process of integration and development of expertise.

The most important quality of highly effective learners is that they are always ready to get help and seek support. As a nursing student you entered your practicum with a rich background of life experiences and thinking skills based on daily living activities. In a sense, you are also building on a source of expertise. By acknowledging what you know and do not know and understanding there are many situations with no right answer, you are developing thinking skills. You are thinking about what to learn and how you learn. Asking for assistance and advice when needed from your instructor is an excellent strategy for analyzing the variety of situations you will encounter in practice.

Creating a learning environment in the agencies and institutions in which you practice is a significant element of integrating knowledge and thinking skills. This means you must get and seek help using multiple sources of expertise. Begin by developing a partnership with your practicum instructor who is your primary source of expertise throughout your clinical rotation. But others, such as peers, experienced nurses, other health-care providers, and your clients, will also prove to be immeasurable sources of help.

Through supervision, your instructor provides you—a novice nurse—with the opportunity to observe, do, and experience in a critically thoughtful way. Learning and getting the most from supervision requires you to make a commitment to active participation with your practicum instructor. Active participation begins with communicating assertively and responsibly with your instructor.

A Helping Relationship

Supervision is a unique helping relationship between a nursing student and an experienced nurse. As a nursing student, supervision offers you both an affirmation and a challenge to your developing nursing practice. It helps you reflect on and critically think about the application of thinking and doing in the nursing process. As a beginning nurse, it is also a way to ensure safe, quality care for your clients. Your practicum instructor provides a supportive context where you can gain and access knowledge for safe and competent practice.

The supervisory relationship between you and your practicum instructor can be a special form of help and support during the clinical rotation. Instructors often serve as influential mentors, coaches, friends, and outstanding role models for acquiring professional competence. Active learning occurs only as you draw on the many resources you'll need as a nurse.

✎ THE SUPERVISORY EXPERIENCE

In order to derive the most from your practica instructors, you will need to know what to expect from them. Your instructors can be expected to help you develop and enhance your professional skills, increase your self-understanding, and promote your learning in countless ways. You can also expect to develop a partnership in learning with your instructors. These relationships usually will be time limited for a specific practicum.

As a student, the most important factor you need to understand at this point in your education is that you can be both a vulnerable learner and competent beginning nurse. Nursing students can expect instructors to help them in four areas: (1) to gain clinical competence; (2) to develop professional confidence and independence; (3) to improve self-awareness; and (4) to acquire theoretical and practice knowledge. With these goals in mind it is reasonable to expect that clinical rotation is a time to *ask questions, explore alternatives,* and to jointly *seek solutions.*

Asking Questions

Asking questions is an important consultative process in acquiring professional competence and integrating content knowledge and thinking. Through asking questions you assume an active role in your learning and enhance the retention of concepts. Asking focused questions is relevant to validating your thinking about issues or checking out approaches to client situations. It is a meaningful way to get help or feedback on your performance. Asking questions is also a communication skill that is potentially critical to the lives of clients in distress. As a beginning nurse your content knowledge will increase each time you ask questions, engage in discussions, and understand what impact your values and beliefs have on your nursing practice.

When and *how* you ask questions is also consequential. Asking questions and seeking information in a timely manner is related to safety issues. Your judgement in various situations must be sound. Therefore, seeking information by asking questions for clarification and validation is related to responsible nursing actions. How you ask a question affects the quality of information you will receive. By asking questions, you develop or establish a mutual problem-solving process with your practicum instructor.

Understanding and applying good communication skills in nursing practice is fundamental to becoming an expert nurse. For example, a nursing student may need to collaborate with other experts such as physiotherapists, social workers, speech therapists, teachers, or parents regarding aspects of client management and treatment coordination. When and how you ask questions will set the stage for various interactions in your practicum with clients, physicians, nurses, and others.

Start with what you know, then ask questions. The more you question the more you learn. If you think you know what to do but are not sure, asking validation questions is a useful technique. That way you have the opportunity to test out your developing clinical judgements and your instructor gets a better idea of how you are progressing in applying theory to practice. Validation questions may take the form of "May I check this out with you? I think I should . . . because . . ."

Exploring Alternative Thinking

Concerned students actively explore alternative ways of thinking about practice and practice situations. Each time that you reflect on your nursing practice you are learning values, beliefs, and expectations essential to the caring process. You are also acquiring professional behaviors. When you reflect on some aspect of your practice, you begin to engage in critical thinking. Reflection is about knowing how you think. Recalling the practice moment allows you to examine the patterns of practice you are engaging in and helps you challenge the way you thought about the practice. Ask yourself if there are alternative ways of doing or thinking about that segment of practice.

Seeking Solutions

Seeking solutions requires you constantly to challenge your intellectual knowledge and interpersonal and technical skills. It requires an examination of your practice paradigms

Notes

and personal knowledge. This process includes looking at assumptions and expectations you have of yourself and others. It means that you will critically appraise the effect of values, beliefs, and expectations on nursing care and your professional behaviors all of which shape your practice outcomes. As a nursing student you will need to challenge yourself in complex and high-risk practice situations with new and different questions. Each time you engage in such inquiries, new ideas and creative thoughts can emerge. Knowing how you think about the practice situation will assist in determining what has been most helpful to you in your learning and what has been least helpful. Reflection is about discovering your being and becoming a competent nurse.

Learning through supervision is a continuous process of self-exploration and change, where you develop reasoning and decision-making skills for competent and safe practice. An effective supervisory partnership leads to untold benefits—it turns the novice learner into an informed learner, the novice nurse into a great nurse.

Learning about Connections

Learning is also about making connections. You will use your practica instructors on an ongoing basis for sources on aspects of practice and professional skill acquisition, technical assistance, special information for client care, and conflict resolution and values issues. You and your instructors will continuously appraise your performance from many perspectives.

Access to your instructors may be associated with regularly scheduled interview times as well as informal opportunities to seek assistance. If your instructors are to be helpful, it is important to examine your reasons for wanting to engage their time. Knowledge and self-evaluation needs must be connected and clearly identified. Preparation for your interview with an instructor is important. Some pre-interview considerations might be:

- What do I need help with?
- What further experiences do I need?
- What am I struggling with?
- How is my progress going in terms of my learning plan?
- How do I evaluate my learning based on my practice experiences?
- May we discuss my personal impressions, reactions, and experiences.

Perceptive Perceptions.   There are specific practice indications for accessing your practicum instructor. Immediate supervision or consultation should be obtained when there are sudden unexpected changes in clients being served. This may include deterioration in status, problems that emerge that were not apparent initially, or when there are issues of safety and protection (medication error). Changes in your ability to carry out expected care also need to be reported promptly (e.g., onset of a migraine headache, family emergency, etc.).

If you are in a preceptored practicum, you preceptor and your institution need to be informed of sick time prior to the onset of your scheduled shift. Acute distress on your part about your ability to cope, to meet objectives, or to maintain positive relationships with agency staff, your preceptor, or peers warrants seeking out an earlier meeting with your instructor. As a student, you need to realize such situations require early or immediate attention. Specific issues should not be reserved until the next scheduled meeting with your instructor.

Paradigms and Personal Knowledge

Problem solving involves a unique mixture of personal knowledge, past concrete situations, individual preferences, and cognitive characteristics and paradigms. These qualities appear to vary considerably among nursing students given the same practical knowledge and unrefined content knowledge (Rogers & Thomlison, 1996). Good problem solving is built upon good descriptions of practice issues. This determines the type of support and understanding you need from your practicum instructor.

Qualities such as your belief systems about self, cases, and assignments will center on concerns stated as, "I don't know what to do with this client" or "How do I go about doing it?" and "I am afraid my client will know I don't know what to do" or "I don't like my client." You need to know that these are normal anxieties of students. These matters translate into concerns that can also be stated as, "I don't know what to do if my instructor realizes I am not helping this person" or "I am afraid my instructor will know I don't know what to do with my client." It is important to share these thoughts with your instructor in the best interests of yourself and clients. As a nursing student, it is natural you are concerned about competence or poor evaluations. The role and focus of your practicum instructor is on the complex task of helping you apply thinking and doing in the nursing process to clients in the clinical setting.

Assumptions and Expectations.   You and your practicum instructor will probe for the assumptions and expectations underlying the assessment and interventions in the practice situation. Narrative accounts of a practice situation are shared and examined in supervision. You will be testing the thinking underlying your practice decisions. Often this will raise new questions and generate new understandings of situations. Reflecting on and discussing the practice of similar and dissimilar client situations, you will learn to expect a certain course of events without ever formally stating those expectations. Sharing of case experiences permits them to be systematically studied and extended or refined for application to other practice situations. Assumptions, expectations, practice patterns, and themes emerge as you learn about practice situations with your practicum instructor. Establishing an environment of safety and trust between you and your instructor is necessary.

SUPERVISION—THE PROCESS

Supervision is the primary process by which nursing students learn to practice competently and safely. It proceeds within a framework shaped by the beginning, middle, and end phases of a dynamic supervisory relationship. Supervision is a give-and-take process that allows understanding to happen. The main tasks and responsibilities of instructors are teaching, supporting, educating, and administrating. Your instructor is there to help you access what you know and what you need to know. You don't need to memorize everything in the textbooks; you just need to know how to find what is in them. This is where your instructor becomes a unique source for making sense of information and helping improve your understanding.

Supervision is essentially the place where you will tell your practicum instructor your practice story, explanations, or reactions to what you are learning and doing. Different supervision activities promote cognitive, affective, and functional learning. Besides direct observation, the agenda or content of supervision may take written and verbal formats. Tapes, didactic discussion, role plays, journals or logs, simulations, case studies, process recordings, and joint work are also activities that form the content of supervision. From these activities, experiences and expectations are clarified and a shared meaning of practice is determined between you and your instructor.

Notes

Supervision goals are dependent on your learning outcomes, the demands of your nursing education program, the opportunities within the clinical practicum, and, to some degree, the orientation of your instructor. Your goals may include skill development, professional growth, self-awareness, and application of theory to a variety of clinical situations. You also will be expected to meet the administrative requirements of the clinical setting. Supervision is thus a type of accountability contract that is explicitly discussed so that both you and your practicum instructor understand what is expected from the process.

Form and Function

The dictionary states the intention of supervision is ". . . to oversee, direct, or manage work, or workers" (Nuefeldt & Guralnik, 1988, p. 1345). Supervision is a dynamic process that assists you to think critically about nursing activities, exploring them from both a personal and nursing perspective. By knowing how you think about your practice activities, you are able to explore, develop, and enhance skills necessary for becoming a great nurse. You learn to build on your existing thinking style to refine and develop your nursing skills and capacities while providing quality nursing care to your clients. Although supervision has an educational focus, you will also learn about yourself in relation to the clinical setting. Educational components of supervision are oriented toward professional and clinical concerns, while management components of your practice are oriented toward policy, practices, and accountability in the setting.

Separating personal and professional issues may be difficult at times. Working with your clients will evoke personal issues for you. These issues must be clearly separated from professional practice decisions. Supervision is not therapy by choice and purpose, and your instructor is not your therapist. If you do need help to work through personal issues triggered by clinical practice, seek out appropriate professional help. Most educational institutions have arrangements for student counseling.

You will find that your practica instructors are flexible, amicable, and approachable, as well as models of the professional qualities of genuineness and congruence (Baird, 1996; Kaiser, 1997; Thomlison, et al., 1996). In addition, you can expect the following elements of supervision:

- **Expectations**—Your instructors will be available for interviews to discuss your unique learning needs and wants. They will expect you to approach them for assistance as needed, even apart from your formal interviews. You should be provided with information on preferred means of communication, such as phone number, e-mail, etc., as well as emergency contact plans, especially if you are in a practicum setting in which the instructor is not present and the hours go beyond usual office hours for your nursing program office.

- **Planning**—Your instructors will plan your clinical assignments. They will balance your assignments so that your cases are both challenging in terms of learning new skills and relevant to your level of competence, with provision for review and integration as well.

- **Modeling**—Your instructors should be role models for you. Observe their professional behavior and management of different situations—from direct clinical practice to conflict resolution. Your instructors will model impeccable professional behaviors while assisting you with learning, supporting, and provide practice behaviors that reflect organizational skills and model elements of authority, trust, and sharing.

- **Feedback**—You can expect your instructors to regularly provide clear, frequent, timely, and relevant feedback about your performance. Feedback will balance your strengths with your vulnerabilities. Confident nursing students ask for feedback and comments as a primary function of their learning.

Supervision provides useful observations, suggestions, ideas, reflections, and directions for novice nurses to learn about the nursing process. From supervision, you will learn about the impact of the environmental, client, and personal factors that affect how nurses provide care. You will have numerous learner requirements to master, but you should demonstrate confidence and be open to your instructors' questioning and analysis of your practice. Your instructors are there to help you view alternative positions about practice cases, projects, or other assignments. Supervision is a complex dynamic process occurring within a specific context for a specific purpose, and it can take various forms.

Practical Matters

There is also a need to tend to practical matters in supervision. When and how often will you interact with your instructor? What do you need to prepare in advance? What portion of the time will be spent on case discussions, specific clinical topics or skills, self-evaluation, professional issues? How are your learning objectives to be demonstrated and evaluated? Are you expected to take the lead or will your instructor? Clarifying the practical matters of supervision helps you manage and shape the results of your learning.

In the instructor-led format, instructors will usually take the lead in questioning you about what you learned preparing for each clinical day, what you see as the priorities of care, and so on. Sometimes they will quiz you about your understanding of the relevant pathophysiology and diagnostic tests or the medications you will be administering. Be prepared to explain what you know and hypothesize. This is excellent preparation for other clinical practice situations in which you will need to succinctly describe pertinent information and relate it to client situation. This type of quizzing often happens at the beginning of the clinical day for two reasons:

1. Your instructors need to be able to quickly appraise your level of knowledge and planning to determine how they will divide time among the students in your group. (Note: The amount of time the instructor spends with you in direct observation also depends on the complexity of the client care situation.)

2. You have this short opportunity to clarify things you found confusing as you did your preparation, especially those things that have immediate implications for the care you provide. Other questions that are more applicable to furthering your own understanding may need to wait until later in the clinical day when you both have more time available, or for a postconference or subsequent meeting.

In the preceptored format, you will probably have more responsibility for initiating meetings with your instructor, organizing three-way evaluation interviews with your preceptor, and establishing the agenda for such meetings. This, too, is part of your learning.

Your instructors will assist you to understand what you know, as well as what you do not know. Learning is a complex function and each student has a preferred approach. Your practicum instructor will be able to teach some aspects of practice, while other components must be learned experientially. Most of all, both of you need to be involved, committed, and interested in the challenges your clients present. To a certain extent, both you and your instructors are learners, learning from each other and each new clinical practice experience.

Supervision Approaches

Supervision occurs in many different formats, but in general nursing students tend to be supervised in a tutor model—in one-to-one or group forms. Depending on the type of setting and the nursing education program, both approaches and other formats such as direct observation (live supervision), or team supervision, may also be offered to you. Summaries of these approaches follow.

Individual Tutor Model. In the individual model of supervision, one nursing student and one practicum nurse instructor meet regularly for a planned meeting that is educationally focused. Your task as a student is to develop critical thinking skills by examining your clinical practice. You need to be open and honest about your practice, and share your feelings, thoughts, and struggles as you strive to understand the practice context. Your responses to authority, power, and clinical approaches to clients are important aspects for discussion and evaluation.

The most typical activity in one-to-one supervision is case discussion, where information about the practice situation is presented to the practicum instructor. This approach will appeal to you if you are a concrete, converger learner and require practical information. Didactic approaches, however, do not address the challenging aspects of reflection and self-exploration styles of learning. Case discussions involve describing your experience with a client, problem, or situation. Usually students identify elements of the case experience and analyze why things happened as they did to discover causes, usefulness, and applicability of what was learned from the contact. Discussion with the practicum instructor teaches you to generalize content knowledge and skills acquired in the specific situation to other clinical situations.

Group Supervision. Group supervision is also an effective approach for students to develop clinical expertise and skills, obtain moral support, and develop self-confidence and awareness. Some students may prefer the group context to the individual tutor model for learning, but most will benefit from settings that provide for teaching, learning, and supporting processes to be balanced in individual and group structures.

Direct Observation. Direct observation is an excellent technique for developing clinical skills because it generates immediate feedback. Your practicum instructor or peers observe you during actual clinical practice. Sometimes your practicum instructor will choose to observe (e.g., doing a dressing change), giving you the opportunity to manage the entire situation and then debrief later. Often your instructor will be a participant observer working with you in managing an episode of patient care (e.g., suctioning a patient's tracheotomy). Even in this situation, debriefing will need to be scheduled later because it would be inappropriate to do a lot of teaching in front of the patient in most situations.

Direct observation is sometimes referred to as live supervision, especially when used in interdisciplinary and family therapy settings. This form of supervision involves performing, monitoring, or suggesting various interventions about dynamics during the actual practice, usually with a family. Your practicum instructor and others watch and listen usually from behind an observation window. Direct or immediate feedback is given to the student in the interviewing room through a variety of communication devices, such as telephone, bug-in-the-ear, notes, or other interventions. The benefits of direct observation are substantial. Immediate corrective feedback is the strongest advantage. Case dynamics are immediately apparent and prompt feedback on performance is available, and a multidimensional perspective is brought to the case analysis. There is greater opportunity for enhancing competence and personal development and students are more likely to integrate new learning in this clinical approach.

🐚 PREPARING FOR CLINICAL DAYS

Most students report learning more from their clinical practice experiences than they do from their classroom experiences. Clinical practice is the "real world" and no amount of course work and lab simulations can actually prepare you for it. Most students anxiously look forward to clinical. After all, this is the reason you chose the field of nursing. When the day finally comes for you to go to your first clinical practice setting, you will probably find yourself with mixed feelings of enthusiasm, anxiety, fear, and uncertainty, perhaps even hoping it is postponed. It begins to dawn on you that you are not ready to practice on "real clients." You are discovering what you know and what you don't know at this point in your nursing education. You realize it may not be the same as reading about a condition in a textbook; it is going to be more complex. Your stress and anxiety are not unique. All students in the helping professions who are about to begin their practicum experience stress, self-doubt, and anxiety. Although it is likely your feelings about getting started in clinical will not diminish until you are actually there and doing it, there are few suggestions to manage your stress before it manages you.

Getting started in your practicum is not always predictable or comfortable and each new practicum brings its own set of uncertainties. The difference is that you will have more skills to fall back on. As one second-year student said, "In my first practicum I didn't even know how to help an elderly lady get out of bed. Now I know I can do that and take her blood pressure too!"

Before You Begin

Before you start clinical practice, you need to realize that you are a student and the practicum is different from the classroom. It is normal for students not to comprehend completely how theory fits into practice at this point in their education. Your practicum instructor will focus on what you can do. *What you know* emerges from the clinical situations you encounter as well as your learning through supervision. You already have a great deal of content knowledge and thinking skills. Remember all the exams and papers you passed? At first, the knowledge and skills necessary for clinical practice may look and feel different from what you were expecting or reading about in your textbook. It is what you do with this knowledge and how you relate the knowledge and facts to the situations you encounter that will be important. Practicum and classroom instructors recognize there is a gap initially for students as they move into practice.

Students encounter quite different client and learning situations during practica. There is no specific text to prepare you for that moment at this stage of your professional development (although this book hopes to assist in this process). To start off in the right directions, experts suggest the following:

🐚 Use honest, clear communication skills and interactions.

🐚 Be flexible in attitude and manner.

🐚 Expect that clinical is going to be different.

🐚 Be open about what you need and want to learn.

🐚 Expect the unexpected.

🐚 Don't forget, you are there to learn.

🐚 Ask questions and seek assistance.

🐚 Build on what you know.

Notes

After all, you are a student and students are not expected to know everything. Asking questions about what you do not yet know will put you in good standing with those in the clinical setting. You will be given an opportunity to try new skills. You will have successes and perhaps some failures, yet both situations provide a wealth of learning. Above all, acknowledging that you want to learn will result in rapid gains in learning.

The Night Before

Students often experience sleepless nights before clinical practica, worrying about many things. "What will my client be like?" "What if my client needs medications and I mess it up?" "What if I harm a client because I don't remember all the procedures for doing an injection?" "What if my client doesn't want a nursing student?" What if the staff doesn't like me?" These are a few of the thoughts students have before clinical. It does seem that some anxiety and self-doubt are universal nursing student worries. Some of the distress may have a reality base, but most of it does not. Doubts about your capabilities create considerable stress. We repeat—you are not required to know everything as a student. You are, however, required to be a concerned learner and develop confidence in yourself and developing skills.

A sense of confidence is the best coping method you can bring forward at this stage. Confident students are much more likely to convey a "can-do" attitude to their clients, who will then be less apprehensive when you are not sure about doing a procedure. Nursing students who have a solid grasp of clinical expectations and who regularly adhere to them will fare just fine. Prepared students know their client priorities and implement decision-making skills for the client's health. Do you understand when you are doing too little or too much? Setting fear and anxiety aside, a positive attitude will go a long way for you, your clients, and your coworkers. Students who like what they do also feel confident and thereby convey hope and respect in client situations. Asking for assistance is the best support and coping strategy to help allay fears and develop confidence.

Unfortunately, your sleepless nights may continue right up until graduation. Remember your classes on the ways to lower your blood pressure and anxiety with relaxation techniques? Now may be the time to practice them.

Getting There

There are also some practical aspects of getting started in your practicum. Be sure you know where you are going and how to get there. How long will it take you? Do you need to take books? If so, find out which ones. Do you need a lunch? Do you have the correct names, addresses, and room locations? Have you written down names that you need to remember? Take the notepad with you. Will you be assigned a locker? A little advance planning, questioning, and preparation can allay many basic organizational anxieties.

Here are some tips to help you survive the first few days.

- Get a checklist from your coordinator with pertinent names, locations, and details for getting to practicum.
- Do a "dry run" to the practicum—going to see where you'll be before the first day is calming.
- Relax; remember, you won't be the only student feeling anxious.
- Use common sense in planning to get there.
- Meet with your instructor in advance to get helpful information about getting to your clinical practicum and questions on your mind.

Making the Most of It

Notes

Enthusiasm and the right attitude are two key survival strategies to a successful practicum. One of the most stressful issues for nursing students is feeling that you cannot make a mistake. You learn in the classroom that you are obligated to obtain all necessary skills and attitudes and to make no mistakes. Nevertheless, you are a student, a learner, and as a learner you have a right to make mistakes as part of the problem-solving process. It is important, however, to distinguish between careless mistakes and mistakes resulting from false reasoning or insufficient data. If you see or hear something you do not understand, ask someone or your practicum instructor. In this way you will discover the facts and feel more confident applying them. As the saying goes, "It is better to ask a dumb question than make a dumb mistake." Besides there are very few "dumb" questions. Most importantly, learn from your mistakes.

Fear of making a medication error haunts most students. If that occurs, report the error *without delay* as soon as you realize it has occurred. Immediate action may save a life. Even if the error is not that serious, it is to your advantage to show that you are conscientious in recognizing and reporting what you have done wrong. Learn why you were wrong or made an error. Make the most of the situation by being open and enthusiastic about the learning process. Learn what you know, and what you need to know. Discuss this with your practicum instructor. Again, remember you do have knowledge, now draw on ways of using that knowledge.

Afterwards

Paying attention to one's emotional and physical self-care is an important component each day you are in clinical. You will probably experience varying emotions and reactions to the day-to-day experiences of the practicum, whether it is about your clients, your peers, yourself, or practicum instructor or even the setting itself. Self-care can go a long way to helping you cope during practicum. Monitoring stress in yourself is a key to your well-being. Relaxation and fun activities need to be considered. Discussing the day with a spouse or partner is not always possible or helpful; nor is it always *ethical*. Keeping a record of your thoughts, experiences, and reactions to the various events and situations you are encountering can help you work out issues. In this way, you will also begin to see yourself in a different light and understand the ways you handle yourself and activities. Your journal is a way to capture your thoughts, feelings, ideas, and discoveries. You are now well on your way to getting started and discovering the joys of learning through supervision.

❧ SUMMARY

- Be open to learning, ask questions, and regularly seek consultation and collaborations.
- There is a wide range of learning styles.
- Learning is a systematic and collaborative strategy between a nursing student and practicum instructor.
- Supervision promotes clinical competence, develops professional confidence and independence, improves self-awareness, and helps you acquire theoretical and practice knowledge.
- The practicum is a potentially stressful experience, so taking care of yourself is essential to your well-being and that of your client.

❧ Becoming a nurse is a decision to accept and seek ongoing supervision as an essential part of learning for your entire professional career.

Supervision prepares the novice nurse to become an expert nurse and more specifically, a caring and competent nurse.

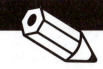

LEARNING TOOL 5.1

Active Learning

LEARNING FOCUS: Values Exploration

Effective learners, no matter what their preferred learning style, are motivated to be lifelong learners. Knowledge is more than memorized information. This exercise will provide you with an opportunity to examine some of your attitudes and assumptions about learning.

STUDENT ACTION

For each of the following statements, place a mark along the line to indicate the amount or frequency with which you demonstrate these attitudes and skills when you are in a learning situation.

Never_____ Always
Question what you read.

Never_____ Always
Summarize points while reading.

Never_____ Always
Consider the context or situation.

Never_____ Always
Consider alternative explanations.

Never_____ Always
Think of specific examples for general statements.

Never_____ Always
Question the obvious.

Never_____ Always
Critically evaluate assumptions.

Never_____ Always
Relate concepts to everyday experience.

Never_____ Always
Relate new concepts to previous learning.

Never_____ Always
Look for evidence to support conclusions.

Never_____ Always
Examine the logic used.

Never_____ Always
Ask for help.

NOTES ON USE

Student Use.   This exercise gives you a chance to extend and build upon your learning style. To be a lifelong learner you need to take an active rather than a "couch potato" approach to your education. This is as true for learning to ski or learning to incorporate regular exercise into your already busy day.

Instructor Use.   For each of the statements ask students to describe situations where this attitude about learning applies or doesn't apply. Have the class develop a list of common fallacies arising from these situations. Highlight the relevance of different ways of learning and how they affect practice decisions. Develop indicators or guidelines for each learning situation to assist students in checking out their assumptions and basis for their knowledge. This encourages students to become critical thinkers. Give illustrations from your learning and practice experiences.

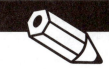

LEARNING TOOL 5.2

My Thinking Style

LEARNING FOCUS: Knowledge Building

Learning is about making connections. An important connection to make involves understanding your preferred ways of learning. This exercise will give you an opportunity to reflect upon your preferences for certain ways or styles of learning, including how you prefer to learn in both formal and informal situations. It may be helpful for you to reread the sections in this chapter or another source on categories of learning styles. Remember that you may see aspects of yourself in more than one style, but you will have a natural or developed preferred way of learning and thinking.

STUDENT ACTION

In this exercise you are asked to (1) describe an example from your own experience that closely resembles each scenario; and (2) write suggestions for changing how each learning scenario was structured to be more conducive to your preferred learning style.

1. The instructor gave a careful explanation of what the lecture would entail. At the end of each section, she summarized the most important points and gave specific, practical examples. The time went quickly even though there was no break or small group interaction.

    Your Example:

    Suggested Changes:

2. The instructor asked the nursing student to explain what he would have done with the patient in terms of major concepts and ideas of the nursing process.

    Your Example:

    Suggested Changes:

3. During the lunch break, two nurses were overheard talking about what they had learned from the case rounds about a young person with HIV and AIDS.

Your Example:

Suggested Changes:

4. The instructor used the image of a learning toolbox with interests, capabilities, experiences, and feelings as sides of the toolbox.

Your Example:

Suggested Changes:

NOTES ON USE

Student Use.   You can learn a great deal about yourself by reflecting on learning situations in which you feel very comfortable, excited, bored, or frustrated. These feelings may indicate that the learning is presented in a way that is compatible with your preferred ways of learning or quite opposite to your preference. You can extend your learning from this exercise by considering two scenarios and then comparing them. First, think of a formal learning situation in which you felt bored or frustrated. Consider what it was about the style of presentation or situation that led to these feelings. Now, do the same for a formal learning situation in which your feelings were very positive and identify elements of the situation or presentation that contributed to these positive feelings. Compare and contrast the two scenarios you have just reflected upon. If you do this across a number of learning situations you will come to identify elements of learning that fit with your preferred ways and those that do not fit.

Instructor Use.   Have students develop a list for each situation based on the class responses and organize the responses by preferred learning approach. Discuss the various ways that each suggestion enhances learning. Emphasize individual needs for understanding and doing. Make sure students share the various approaches to learning each situation.

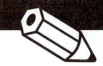

LEARNING TOOL 5.3

Mapping Decision Making

LEARNING FOCUS: Critical Thinking Enhancement

This exercise explores the decision-making process you use in both everyday and clinical situations.

STUDENT ACTIONS

Think about a decision that you need to make or have recently made. It does not need to be a life-altering decision, but it would be best if it was important enough to be carefully considered. Create a decision map using the following categories. Some suggestions of questions to ask yourself have been supplied.

1. **Background Information**
   What makes this decision necessary? What are the "facts"? Is the information that I have reliable? Does it come from reliable sources? What is responsible for the problem?

2. **Decision Options**
   What are my options? How will I decide which are best? What values of mine come into play when I think about each option? What are the consequences of each option? How do I weigh the consequences for me and for others?

3. **Best Option**
   Which option do I consider to be the best?

4. **From Option to Action**
   How can I carry the best option out?

Now apply the same process to a nursing decision that you had to or might need to make in your current clinical practicum.

1. **Background Information**
   What makes this decision necessary? What are the "facts"? Is the information that I have reliable? Does it come from reliable sources? What is responsible for the problem?

LEARNING TOOL 5.3 continued

2. **Decision Options**

   What are my options? How will I decide which are best? What values of mine come into play when I think about each option? What are the consequences of each option? How do I weigh the consequences for me and for others?

3. **Best Option**

   Which option do I consider to be the best?

4. **From Option to Action**

   How can I carry the best option out?

NOTES ON USE

Student Use.   There is a lot of leeway for deciding how you complete this exercise, which may be more or less comfortable for you. Take note of your feelings when doing this or any of the exercises. This is information about yourself and your preferred ways of doing things. You can learn a lot from others, so be willing to share your process with them.

Instructor Use.   This exercise gives students a way to test the thinking underlying their practice decisions. You might suggest a visual representation of the decision process through a decision tree. This might be helpful for more concrete learners. Provide an example that you had to make recently.

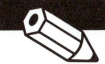

LEARNING TOOL 5.4

Decision Making in Practice

LEARNING FOCUS: Application Enhancement

In making decisions, we all use cues from the situation to aid us in the process of deciding. Expert nurses make context-dependent judgements, while more novice nurses tend to rely on context-free rules to guide decisions. No matter where you are along the continuum from novice to expert, use this exercise to expand the number of factors you utilize in decision making.

STUDENT ACTION

Read and then reread the following case. Answer the questions and complete the tasks that follow.

> *Your learning assignment for the morning is to prepare a patient for a day surgery procedure. Mr. Montoya, a 54-year-old janitor and father of five children, is scheduled for a hemorrhoidectomy at 0900. On greeting Mr. Montoya in the waiting area you notice that he is a small, thin man, somewhat stooped, and looking older than his stated age. His wife and eldest son are sitting with him, looking quite anxious. Mr. Montoya says very little as you show him to his room. After leaving him for a few moments to get into his hospital gown, Mrs. Montoya confides in you that her husband has not been taking his "blood pressure and water pills" because they make him "sick". She tells you that he has never been in hospital before and is very frightened about "being put to sleep". You carefully take his vital signs and record them on the preoperative assessment form: BP 154/98, P88, R 22, T 96.8° F. He assures you that he has had nothing to eat this morning, just his usual coffee and cigarette. He doesn't think he is allergic to anything, but tells you he got a bad rash one time after the doctor taped up his broken finger. As you finish the preoperative assessment form and checklist he asks you how long he'll have to be off work. Otherwise he has no questions about his surgery.*

1. What are your hunches about this case and your course of action?

2. What would your decision for action be?

3. What factors did you utilize in coming to a decision?

4. What factors were extraneous to your decision?

5. Rank the factors you used in order from most important to least important.

6. How were your hunches related to the choice and ranking of the cues or factors considered in your decision?

7. Ask an experienced nurse to read the case and give you a glimpse into his or her thinking and decision-making process. Note the similarities and differences in how you thought about the case.

NOTES ON USE

Student Use.   Don't be discouraged by any differences between yourself and the experienced nurse with whom you consult. You're learning—that's why they call you a nursing student!

Instructor Use.   Students should complete their responses to the case independently. Then, form students into small groups to discuss their responses. Have the groups report what they consider the best responses to the case. Have the class share and discuss the group responses.

LEARNING TOOL 5.5

Helping Relationships That Help

JOURNAL FOCUS

The quality of your relationships with professionals who are assigned to assist you in your learning can facilitate or hinder that learning. Some persons come closer to what you expect or need in a learning situation than do others. This exercise will provide you with an opportunity to explore some of your perceptions and expectations of those who are important in your learning process.

STUDENT ACTION

Choose one professional relationship, such as instructor or preceptor, on which to reflect. Assess the relationship in terms of the following dimensions and qualities.

Place a mark along the line to indicate how you perceive the relationship.

Very Interested _____ Not Interested

Interest in helping me to learn.

Very Open _____ Not Open

Open to questions.

Very Willing _____ Not Willing

Gives sufficient time to students.

Very Interested _____ Not Interested

Interest in helping me to think.

Very Able _____ Not Able

Able to orient students to nursing setting.

Assess the current quality of the relationship between yourself and the professional you chose for the previous section. Again, mark where along the line between the two dichotomies you perceive your relationship to be.

Congenial _____ Conflictual

Trusting _____ Mistrustful

Cooperative _____ Competitive

Sluggish _____ Animated

Satisfactory _____ Frustrating

Cohesive _____ Divisive

POSITIVE STATEMENTS ABOUT ME

Remember, at the end of each journal entry you are to draw out from your reflections and journal writing positive statements you can make about yourself. Make each statement an "I" statement.

NOTES ON USE

Student Use.   After completing your perceptions of the dimensions and quality of the professional relationship, write about your reflections in the journal. Try to use "I" statements to describe the relationship based on your assessment of the exercise.

Instructor Use.   Assist students to think about and recognize where they can take responsibility for their learning and how to use the professional relationships. This exercise will encourage students to be aware of what they know and don't know, how to be proactive in their preferred approach, and how others differ from them. Is there another way of thinking about this situation? Self-criticism helps students discover and correct faulty perceptions about learning and decision making.

6

Logging Life's Ups and Downs

JOURNAL THOUGHT

Write down everything, leave nothing standing. Experiences, meanings, theories, and con-cepts. All are relevant. . . . I've learned about personal views on health to a great extent. In many cases, I've discovered insights and meanings I never knew I had. The journal really has been beneficial. It's encouraged me to explore my beliefs, examine them for meanings, and question the origin of these values.

NURSING STUDENT

This chapter is about recording what is happening during your clinical rotation. Writing assists you to focus and reflect on the significance of activities or events as they relate to learning to be a nurse. Though you chronicle significant and meaningful events, it is the process of writing that is really important. When writing is organized and directed it is more likely to improve the learning process. The process of critical thinking forms the basis for writing, searching for details of events, formulating themes, and communicating results. Above all, it should be relevant to you and enhance your learning needs. The types of writing and recording discussed in this chapter include journaling, clinical logs, audio and video taping, and a practice portfolio.

JOURNAL WRITING

The journal, or directed diary, is one of the most important tools you have at your disposal to document the events in your clinical rotation. It can be simple or complicated. Above all, it is a tool for learning while you are in school and long after you graduate.

Notes

The journal is an ancient tool that goes back to the tenth century when Japanese ladies of the court used the "pillow book" to reflect on life and love. During the seventeenth century Protestants and Puritans applauded the self-discipline of the diary.

Journaling is somewhat different from keeping a diary. As a journal writer, you will primarily focus on external events related to your learning, thinking, and doing as a nursing student. It is a safe place to raise issues, deal with your fears and concerns, and log life's ups and downs. It is a place where you can be yourself.

WHAT IS A JOURNAL?

A journal is an analytical tool for recording facts, events, and processes. Your journal should include a record of observations, experiences, and the impact of these events on your life. Different processes come into play using the written word rather than the spoken word. It is a form of personal feedback about what you see and hear in your environment.

Starting Your Journal

The secret to journal writing is simply to start. Begin anywhere—with how you feel, with a question, with the best thing that happened today or the worst thing. It does not really matter. What does matter is that you begin to put your thoughts, ideas, and feelings on paper. You are not journaling to become a good writer. It is a purposeful process that helps support the development of particular qualities such as humility, integrity, perseverance, empathy, and self-discipline. As you write, you are able to identify the elements of thought present in a problem or event in the clinical rotation—and you make connections between the elements and the issue or problem at hand. You write to clarify thinking and form a baseline against which to measure change in yourself. It is a forum in which you can ask yourself about many things. Are you comfortable with your communication skills with clients? Do you feel anxious when you change dressings? Do you feel uncomfortable approaching your instructor? Are you proud of your relationship skills with other health-care providers?

You will want to review your journal entries regularly for themes, ideas, and patterns. You will also want to consider what the events mean and how you feel about them. Journaling is a way to organize and summarize thoughts. Some helpful tips for starting a journal follow:

- Be brief.
- Write as much as you need to get your point across.
- Always include one positive statement about your abilities and strengths.
- Don't be concerned about grammar and spelling, unless directed otherwise by your instructor.
- Write using language that will not embarrass you.
- Each time you write appraise your thinking.
- Make daily entries, or at least around each clinical encounter.
- Use any book, but a loose-leaf binder helps you to move pages around for comparisons.
- Reread your entries as a form of feedback.
- Try using different colored pens for various entries: thoughts about your clients, unplanned events, issues, moods, or your achievements, etc.

- Try to keep your journal entries neat.
- A two-column format provides space to return to the entry for later reflection and additions.

Your journal writing involves carefully examining and evaluating beliefs, feelings, and actions. It requires paying attention to the process of reasoning or critical thinking in your writings. Well-reasoned thinking is a creative way to understand your purpose and learn about your learning.

Guidelines for Your Journal

The purpose of journaling is self-assessment and self-improvement. Through journal writing you will discover assumptions, alternative explanations, and biases about yourself as a developing professional nurse. You will also uncover your abilities and strengths from this self-discovery process. Self-assessment is another opportunity to learn. Through your journal entries, you can evaluate processes of nursing and your nursing practice. Ultimately, your journal is evidence of your accomplishments and learning experiences. But each time you write and appraise your thinking you are also helping your clients in valuable ways. Your journal can assist you in planning for safe, quality choices and options for clients as you provide nursing care.

Some guidelines for using your journal effectively include:

- Think in terms of opposites.
- Explore different views from different perspectives.
- Focus on problem finding and problem solving.
- Emphasize understanding.
- Reflect on the language you use.
- Recognize affective influences.
- Recognize attitudes and values associated with cognitive biases.
- Reflect on self-awareness by asking, "What do I believe? Why do I believe that?"
- Identify recurring patterns of interaction.
- Keep your journal in a safe or private place.

Now that you understand the purpose of journaling and writing steps, you are ready to begin to explore ideas, beliefs, and attitudes evident in your writings. Some of the primary activities you will do with your journal writing include reflecting on practice and self, exploring feelings, working through problems, questioning, and thinking critically. This task requires you to be both honest and willing to write with integrity. Remember, client names should never be used, even in your personal journal.

Reflecting

Writing and reflecting are intricately intertwined. In fact, putting pen to paper (or fingers to laptop) is what compels us to reflect. Writing is a learning tool for heightening and refining the process of reflection. Reflection promotes inner or emotional awareness. It is a cognitive process.

The purpose of writing about the events and experiences from your clinical rotation is to think about their meaning for you as a learner and developing professional. The more you become aware of the significance of these practice experiences, the more you are able to tap into your inner strengths and capacities. Your focus should be on your unfolding awareness of self and the meaning, values, and interrelationships you are discovering in your learning experiences as a nursing student. Journal writing generates positive thoughts, provides you with a clearer sense of self, helps you use your strengths to improve your nursing care. Remember to always record one positive thought about your abilities or strengths in each entry.

Exploring Feelings

Logging life's ups and downs gives you an opportunity to explore your feelings about the clinical rotation and your experiences with clients, colleagues, peers, and your supervisor. One helpful technique is to pose questions that provide direction. For example: What frustrates me in my clinical rotation? What frustrates me in working with my client? Why is my learning so stressful? What is my biggest fear in this setting? What aspects of my work accomplishments am I most proud of? What have I excelled at? Questions help you uncover your feelings about many issues. Seeing your thoughts in writing gives you a different perspective and likely provides a balanced view of your successes and challenges. By exploring your feelings about your work, you can gain insights into yourself, your clients, and coworkers, and put the meaning in daily events, activities, and experiences in perspective. Reflecting on your feelings is also a necessary part of professional growth.

Working through Problems

Writing requires you to cluster ideas, develop themes, and organize your thoughts about the problems of your clients and your practice skills. It is a way to work through problems or questions and validate your thoughts and observations. Some techniques that are helpful in addressing problems in the nursing environment include an interpretive approach to the nursing world, practice setting, and caring practices. Writing about your experiences in dealing with a client, and your interpretation of the problems you encountered, allows you to see the factors affecting the nursing process and helps you learn how to incorporate content knowledge with clinical practice. You can also examine alternative approaches to nursing care and stretch your learning and knowledge building along the continuum from novice to expert.

As a nursing student, you can work through problems by organizing or focusing your journal on aspects such as:

- Defining the situation of the client—understand the client from a historical and current view.
- Reacting to the client—what are your perceptual and emotional reactions to the client?
- Viewing the client from a time perspective—project the client into the future and compare the client from the past.
- Examining common meanings of the client's life with yours—what are possible issues that are common or different?
- Writing a narrative of the client's story or journey through illness.
- Writing a narrative about a struggle you had in your life.
- Reflecting on a client's response to a diagnosis.
- Defining expectations of your nursing role in providing care for a client/patient.

The objective of working through nursing problems using a narrative or journal writing approach is to help you increase your skills in recognizing client concerns and assisting in the communication with clients and others. New insights and meanings emerge from examining your responses and the client's responses to caring practices. Learning to connect with your client increases your skills in interpretive listening and understanding. Not only will your active listening skills be enhanced, your analytical and interpretive skills will also develop. Journal writing about practice and problems enables you to hear and interact with your own voice and concerns in a clinical situation Enhancing your thinking skills creates a personal paradigm for nurturing responsibility and accountability in nursing.

Questioning

Journal writing should be organized around concerns even though initially you may not know what these concerns are. Formulate questions about your observations or concerns. Write your questions in the first person. This allows you to personalize and learn from your successes and failures. Your questions and journal responses reveal human meanings and concerns, moral issues, and concrete know-how based on your practice experiences. Your dialogue about practice situations helps develop your self-understanding, improve your performance, and hone your skills of perceiving and responding to your clients' needs.

Critical Thinking

The process of critical thinking forms the basis for writing—searching for detail, formulating patterns, and communicating results. Free from the confines of the classroom and the clinical rotation setting, your journal is a place to think aloud. Here you can open up and explore your thoughts. You can reveal to yourself what you know and what you need to know. You can examine your decision making and see where a care plan lacks clarity. A journal helps you identify where your thinking breaks down. It assists in learning clinical judgement and the critical thinking process. The information that comes from both self-evaluation and client evaluation of outcomes are important aspects of critical thinking about your practice.

Think back over your own development. What are some of the incidents and events that have shaped your desire to help others? What are the stages in your learning as a developing nurse? What is your vision of the ideal nurse? How would you describe yourself in relation to this ideal vision? How does your cultural background affect your care practice? What needs to occur in your practice for you to meet the next stage of learning development? These critical thinking or evaluative questions ask you to make judgements about the quality of your developing work as a nursing student. This, in part, assists you in determining such things as whether you are doing satisfactory nursing care, whether your instructor is aware of your work, and whether you are staying within the parameters of the ethical code of the nursing profession. It also helps you assess what you need to learn in order to work more safely and competently.

❧ CLINICAL LOGS

Other forms of writing and documenting also support your learning. Writing or recording clinical elements of the cases you have been assigned assists you and your client in numerous ways. This form of writing is more objective because you will record events as they happen, as well as what these events or transactions mean to you and how you feel about them. In clinical logs you document processes, activities, and transactions between you and your client, as well as describe and react to the dilemmas of practice posed by your clients and others.

Clinical logs can be reviewed, discussed with your instructor, and analyzed for learning. Confidentiality is, therefore, an important aspect of paradigm case recordings

Notes

and other clinical logging activities. Always remember that names, places, and other identifying data should be changed to protect you and your client.

Paradigm Cases

Writing about a case assignment or real-life practice situations provides a framework for examining your thinking, doing, and knowing. Case analysis, particularly of your failures, can have a powerful influence on your learning. It helps you conceptualize problems and determine more appropriate methods of approaching and thinking about your clients and future clinical situations.

Paradigm cases are cases that stand out for you in some way. A paradigm case is like a diamond. You can examine it from many angles and still find something new, something beautiful. Paradigm cases are about questioning the theory and practice of what helps clients. A paradigm case is helpful in examining your hands-on experiences and reviewing and analyzing your learning style (see Chapter 5).

Select a case from your current practice assignments and write case process notes about a meaningful encounter or transaction that occurred between you and your client. Select a case with special meaning—a case where you made a connection at some level. Write about the case being as descriptive as you can, that is, remembering all of the details. It is important to describe the location and surrounding events, the sights, sounds, and smells and their impact on you, as well as the verbal and nonverbal ways your client presented to you and any other impressions. How did your client react to the environment? Also recall all of your own verbal and nonverbal communications in the interaction. It is important to explore all aspects of the interaction.

Now, use your analytical skills. How did you know what to do in this case—by accident, planning, reading, or by trial and error? Consider how you handled the case. What aspects generated stress for you? What aspects did you handle well? What was your reaction to your nursing tasks and how did you manage them? Analysis of paradigm cases hones critical thinking skills. You should chronicle both your achievements and struggles. In fact, learning is more likely to emerge from the struggles and questions about the case and your practice in that situation.

Using a case for learning requires you to write the information in organized ways that identify significant and meaningful aspects of the case; for example: client's self-presentation, client's mood, nursing student's presentation to client, nursing student's mood, and nature of the encounter. As you describe what each of you said and did, you must also explore whether you could have influenced the process in other ways. For example, what occurred that might have influenced your actions or feelings? What does this mean to your care of the client? In what ways did this case change what you learned about yourself or your client? Summarize the case by identifying how you learned from this situation.

A paradigm case asks you to think carefully about what you did and what you thought about it. Paradigm cases are essential parts of your developing self-awareness and knowledge base. Paradigm cases will help you analyze your achievements toward learning goals, acquisition of psychomotor skills, and developing professional identity as a nurse.

Case Segment Notes

Case notes, or case segment notes, capture a briefer aspect of your learning. Case notes also contribute to client care and the quality of your nursing care, but the focus is on writing about a segment of a piece of practice. In the paradigm case, you record the complete transaction or exchange. In a case segment note, you choose a part of the transaction or event then write about it and analyze it. You will also write verbatim

Notes

about that segment before you begin to analyze the process. Here you may focus on particular features of your learning, for example, your role or skills. In what ways did you show professionalism to your client with Alzheimer's disease? How easily did you manage taking an adolescent's sexual history? Based on part of your interview with the new mom about breast-feeding, how and what would you do differently?

A useful way for you to write and analyze case segment notes follows:

- Describe verbatim a segment of an interview, interaction, or situation.
- Write about the statements you made and those of your client.
- Under a separate heading, identify your feelings about that event during the time of its occurrence.
- Under a separate heading, identify and assess the psychomotor skill used.
- Under a separate heading, what alternative ways of handling the exchange, feeling, or skill would be a preferred response? What aspects of the segment should be done in the same way?

In the same way that journal writing helps you to examine both content and process of your nursing practice, case segment notes help you understand what you are doing, what you are feeling, and what you are thinking. You are using similar tools to assess what you know and what you need to know as you move from novice to expert nurse.

AUDIO- AND VIDEOTAPING

A common technique for capturing case content is taping—either by audio recording or videotaping. Some individuals believe that these technical methods are superior to other forms of collecting information, such as journal writing and clinical logs, for teaching purposes. The use of audio- or videotaping simply provides a different view of content and process and, therefore, is essentially an additional way of learning for those whose preferred approach is more visual and auditory.

Recording Information

Videotaping requires access to equipment and often takes place in a studio-like atmosphere. Therefore, it is not often feasible to videotape a client in certain settings. Videotaping a client or a simulation provides a full recording of an actual exchange, which has certain advantages. Tapes serve as a mirror to accurately reflect your practice and communication skills. Self-confrontation and self-awareness are two benefits you can derive from tapes. The examination of verbal and nonverbal elements of interaction from viewing the tapes assists nursing students to develop and assess content and process. Videotaping a psychomotor skill performed in a clinical or simulated setting lets you analyze the sequence, efficiency of steps, and precision of technique as well as interaction with the client during the procedure.

An alternative to working with videotaping clients is to role-play with other nursing students a situation or interaction about some aspect of your clinical rotation or case assignments. Some things to look for in reviewing videotape include:

- body language and behavior;
- language used and tone of voice;
- speech patterns; and
- degree of comfort in executing a skill or interaction.

Notes

Through taping of clients or role-plays, you learn to understand your reactions, yourself, and specific situations of nursing practice. As you become aware of and are able to understand where you have gaps in learning your practice skills are likely to improve. Videotaping role-plays helps reduce apprehension before you see a client and allows you to practice nursing skills and gain confidence.

The advantage of an audiotape recording is that the recorder is portable and can be taken with you to different locations. While it certainly does not capture the visual aspects for analysis, it does allow you to record your verbal interactions or contacts exactly as they occurred. Many nursing settings and programs have opportunities for students to access both technologies for learning. Remember, if you are taping clients using either form of technology you must seek consent to tape in order to protect your client.

Guidelines for Recording

The following basic guidelines should be observed when audio- and videotaping either a client or role-play situation:

- Practice using the equipment before the actual recording situation.
- Keep taping equipment visible.
- Relax, it is natural to feel somewhat anxious about taping for the first time.
- Nursing students tend to believe clients will not give approval for taping, but clients do readily consent.
- Present the request for being taped in a relaxed manner to the client.
- Always ask for written permission to tape a client. Some agencies require that the client repeat permission to be taped at the beginning of the recording. Do not use client names.
- Fully explain to the client exactly who will be viewing the tape (e.g., you, your instructor, etc.), the purpose of reviewing the tape, and how long the tape will be kept. Include this information in a written consent form.
- You also do not have to tape the full interaction with a client if that is preferable.
- Making a tape available for clients to view or listen to is often a clinically helpful tool in working with a client.
- Store the tape in a safe location, if a client was taped.
- Indicate a time frame for erasing the tape.

THE PRACTICE PORTFOLIO

Documenting your experiences in the form of a practice portfolio has extensive benefits. All nursing students need to have a record of practice accomplishments. Practice records provide an ongoing profile of cases, skills, special projects, and assignments completed during your practicum. The portfolio is useful as a review of progress, but it is also helpful in compiling your strengths and attributes for potential employers, graduate school, registration and licensing requirements, and for evaluative purposes for you and your instructor/preceptor. Your profile will be unique, so there are many ways to set up this record. At the very least, the practice profile should record the following:

1. Case exemplars
2. Self-assessment (see Learning Tools 3.2 and 8.2)
3. Checklist of psychomotor skills attainment

4. Special knowledge acquired
5. Sample assignments completed—illustrate best practices, or review your journal for how you constructed knowledge among cases or between clients
6. Review your course outlines for knowledge acquisition
7. Other illustrations—teaching, coaching, cooperative learning, or mastery of procedures, etc.

The record of your practice portfolio is a summative evaluation of your learning. It can be used from year to year during your nursing education and maintained well into your nursing career. Keeping a practice profile is important and, therefore, you will want to update this portfolio regularly.

CONSTRUCTING AND DECONSTRUCTING INFORMATION

The benefits of journaling, writing case logs, and/or making electronic recordings include discovering better alternatives in nursing care plans, which ultimately enhances the quality of your decision-making skills. All of the forms of writing and analysis discussed allow you as a nursing student to communicate with yourself. Through constructing and deconstructing your experiences and perspectives of nursing care you evolve and improve your understanding of both the content and processes you are using. Your instructor is also a source of help in analyzing these materials, which can assist your learning immensely. The primary purpose in analyzing your work is to improve your responses to clients, thus improving nursing interactions. By rereading your journal and other case recordings, you sort out the facts from your feelings. You bring theory to your practice and you gain knowledge about nursing care and yourself.

Undertake the following tasks as you examine your writings, paradigm cases, or tapings:

- discover patterns;
- reveal themes;
- regroup information;
- differentiate facts from opinions;
- cluster related information; and
- distinguish descriptions from inferences.

To enhance the learning process there are several analytical strategies focused on learning and thinking questions arising from your writings.

Insights and Questions

All of the learning strategies discussed in this chapter help nurture a reflective style to your nursing practice. As a reflective thinker, new insights and questions will emerge in your day-to-day practice. Tracking your activities and describing your thoughts takes a lot of work, but there is a payoff. Your level of sensitivity about yourself will increase as will your self-confidence in your developing abilities as a nurse. The insights derived from analyzing your work will lead to creative nursing approaches and new ideas. Review what you are learning and relate it to your learning goals. For synthesis and integration to occur, students need to understand the content of their practice. Monitoring the type of questions you are writing down can help you determine further theory and content you need to learn.

Notes

Integrating Knowledge with Clinical Practice

Journal writing and the other methods of collecting information about you and your progress during clinical rotation are concerned with moving you beyond a beginner's way of gaining knowledge. Each analysis has a particular framework to connect knowledge with clinical practice. Having knowledge is not sufficient, you need to know how to apply the knowledge appropriately in real-life situations with clients.

Discovering Emerging Patterns.   Integration of theory into practice is the desired outcome of your learning. Integration of learning occurs best when you identify and examine your activities and discover patterns. The factors affecting your practice can be identified by discovering emerging patterns in your work. You may need to modify some aspects of your interactions or activities, while others are patterns you will want to repeat in order to reinforce them. This allows you to identify the positive skills and build on emerging interests and strengths on your journey to expert nurse.

Finding Out More

Constructing or deconstructing information requires nursing students to think about what they are doing in theoretical and practical ways in order to organize their information into usable format for improving care practices. You analyze your work by examining theories, interpretations, and feelings. The analysis helps you frame solutions, rethink approaches, and articulate new goals for learning. Each situation you encounter in clinical rotation presents a unique learning opportunity. Each form of collecting and collating information discussed above will also present a unique approach to your learning and thinking. It is important for you to understand the relevance of the various forms of learning to your overall learning objectives and development. The classic analytical framework of "who, why, when, where, what, and how" are always useful in reaching conclusions about what you are learning in practicum. Organizing information about clients and yourself helps you reach conclusions and determine if you need more information or opportunities.

❧ SUMMARY

Journaling, writing clinical logs, and taping are tools for learning better skills and nursing practice. They help build self-awareness, refine assessment skills, and support your learning to work effectively as a nurse. Keeping a journal and a practice portfolio are key strategies for critical thinking. Analyzing your capabilities brings you along the continuum from novice to expert nurse.

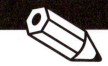

LEARNING TOOL 6.1

In a Different Voice

LEARNING FOCUS: Values Exploration

Each of us has had struggles and difficulties in life. This is something you share with patients/clients. You may not have had the same experience but you have overcome other life struggles. This learning exercise is designed to help you get in touch with some inner resources and strategies that you can use for yourself and to assist others you will meet in clinical situations.

STUDENT ACTION

Choose a situation to describe in which you had to handle criticism from someone—perhaps an instructor or a patient.

1. Write a narrative account of the experience. You may write it in the first person ("I") or in the third person ("she or he"). The latter will give you greater distance from which to view the experience, while the former will put you much more clearly in the action.

2. Now rewrite the narrative using the other person. That is, if you used the first person, now write in the third person or vice versa.

3. Reread the two narratives you have created. Focus on your feelings. What feelings arose while writing and reading the narratives? Were they the same or different depending upon the narrative voice?

LEARNING TOOL 6.1 continued

4. In which voice was it easier to view things from the other person's perspective?

5. Write the narrative of this situation from the perspective of the person who criticized you. Use "I" for that person's voice.

NOTES ON USE

Student Use.   Encountering criticism is never easy, yet it provides us with an opportunity to learn and grow. Putting yourself in the place of the person delivering the criticism may not be easy but it may help you to better understand them. You can practice scenarios with your classmates to help you handle criticism from patients or clients.

Instructor Use.   The scenarios students develop provide an excellent opportunity to discuss and rehearse handling criticism from clients/patients. This would be an appropriate time to collect stories of patient criticisms from their previous or current practica. The group can discuss how the criticism looked from the student's perspective but also what might have been going on for the client. This will help students develop empathy and some important interpersonal skills. Students can reflect on what type of "bedside manner" they want to develop.

LEARNING TOOL 6.2

Seeking Help

LEARNING FOCUS: Knowledge Building

To manage your nursing practica successfully, you must be aware of your personal issues about receiving and seeking help. Your thoughts, feelings, and experiences about asking for and receiving help from others influence how you will relate to clients who need your help.

STUDENT ACTION

You are asked to consider three types of help-seeking situations in this exercise. You will write about your thoughts, feelings, and actions prior to and following your seeking help.

SCENARIO ONE (RECENT SITUATION IN WHICH YOU ASKED FOR AND RECEIVED HELP)

1. Describe the scenario.

2. What were your feelings about asking for help?

3. What were your thoughts about asking for help?

4. What actions were taken in seeking help?

5. What would you do differently the next time?

SCENARIO TWO (RECENT SITUATION IN WHICH YOU ASKED FOR HELP AND HELP WAS NOT GIVEN BY THE PERSON)

1. Describe the scenario.

2. What were your feelings about asking for help and not receiving it?

3. Did you receive no help or just not the help that was useful for you?

4. What were your thoughts about asking for help and not receiving it?

5. What actions were taken in seeking help? What did you do after not receiving help from this person?

6. What would you do differently the next time?

SCENARIO THREE (RECENT SITUATION IN WHICH YOU NEEDED HELP BUT YOU DID NOT ASK OR ASK DIRECTLY FOR HELP)

1. Describe the scenario.

2. What were your feelings about not asking for help?

3. What were your thoughts about not asking for help?

4. What actions were taken instead of seeking help?

5. What would you do differently the next time?

NOTES ON USE

Student Use.   Look at the similarities and differences between your thoughts and feelings in these situations. Reexamine your actions as well. Do you tend to ask directly in some situations but not in others? What is different about these situations? Do you subtly expect people who know you to "read your mind" and anticipate your needs and meanings? Examining the interrelationship between your thoughts, feelings, and actions is based upon cognitive-behavioral theory.

Instructor Use.   You might explore other common thought patterns besides "mind reading," such as all-or-nothing thinking, overgeneralization, mental filter, jumping to conclusions, overlooking the positive, and should statements (Burns, 1980). From case examples, you could help students identify when the nurse or the client might have been using some common thought patterns. These case examples could also be used to identify compassionate responses to patients who may have difficulty asking for help.

LEARNING TOOL 6.3

It's What You Didn't Say

LEARNING FOCUS: Critical Thinking Development

In this exercise you will have a chance to examine the quality of your communication skills through creating several case segment logs. Effective relationship skills are an asset that you will want to cultivate. They enable you to establish rapport with patients/clients, as well as engender the confidence and cooperation of the very people whom you are poised to help.

STUDENT ACTION

The verbatim segment of an interaction may seem tedious, but it can be well worth the effort by uncovering often unspoken and unnoticed aspects of the interaction. Since it is easier to note many aspects of an interaction when you are not a direct participant but more of an observer, watch an interaction between a nurse and a client/patient, then record the following:

1. Write verbatim a small segment of an interview, interaction, or situation that you observed between a client/patient and a health-care professional. The two-column format suggested below is often helpful to keep the interaction straight.

Client Speaking   **Health-care Professional Speaking**

2. Write about how each of the participants influenced the interaction by both verbal and nonverbal aspects of the interaction.

3. Identify your feelings about the events as you observed them happening.

4. Identify aspects of the interaction that you thought went well and would not change, as well as alternative ways of handling the exchange that might have produced a different result.

Now, select a segment of an interaction between yourself and a client/patient. Unless you are experienced at this type of writing, you may want to limit the players in the interaction to you and one client. If you really want to challenge yourself, add one or more persons to the interaction. You can do the recording from memory, but it may be more helpful to decide ahead of time that your next interaction with a particular person will be the focus of your verbatim analysis. Allow yourself time after your interaction to write or to at least make notes for later use.

1. Write your "he said, she said" notes here. *Leave spaces after each statement or question to record further information.*

Client Speaking   **Yourself Speaking**

2. Now, go back over your case segment notes and add to them comments about nonverbal communications—include both your own and the client(s). For example, note tone of voice or posture or even the distance between you and the client.

3. Now, go back and include in the notes the level of awareness you had during the interaction regarding these nonverbal cues. For example, were you aware that your tone of voice raised when you commented on something or that the client got very quiet when the subject of family came up. You can rate your level of awareness at the time using descriptors such as "not aware" or "very aware" or you can rate the level of awareness on a scale from 1 to 9.

4. Attend to the emotional content of the interaction. Look at not only the feelings involved but the intensity of the feelings—yours and the client's. Record these at the appropriate places in the verbatim recording.

5. Read over the following list of relationship skills and note in the segment notes when specific skills were demonstrated. This is only a partial list—please add skills as needed.

Offered empathetic responses.	Listened well.
Asked helpful questions.	Comforted when appropriate.
Offered encouragement.	Accepted compliments or praise.
Conveyed respect.	Offered suggestions.
Considered client feelings.	Accomplished purpose.

6. Which of these relating skills would you like to further develop? How might you strengthen your skill level in these areas?

NOTES ON USE

Student Use.   This exercise deals with the purposeful use of "self" in interactions with your clients. Remember that the purpose of case segment notes is to examine the content ("the what") and process ("the how") of nursing practice. This technique will help you to understand what you are doing, what you are feeling, and what you are thinking. You can use this technique to assess what you know and what you need to know in many nursing situations.

Instructor Use.   This exercise can be a written assignment that you mark, or you can have students exchange and mark each other's assignments. This exercise assesses the use of communication and relationship skills in a given interaction. You can extend this exercise by having students examine a series of interactions to assess how they put these skills into practice in a consistent way and if they can implement these skills across situations.

LEARNING TOOL 6.4

Serendipity in Learning

LEARNING FOCUS: Application Enhancement

During a reflection on a clinical experience with an elderly woman in a nursing home, a nursing student, Susan, connected the objective and subjective viewpoints. She wrote:

> During my reflection on this experience, I realized that by moving my understanding from an objective point of view to a "subjective, lived meaning" I could empathize with her situation better. The objective viewpoint is what I can observe; her behavior, likes and dislikes, moods, and the way she goes about her daily life. By looking at it subjectively, as was discussed in class, I am better able to understand her actions are a result of her lived experience, such as her being at the nursing home and her husband being at home. Transforming our viewpoint from objective to subjective is an excellent way to empathize with the client, and put yourself in their position. Integrating the subjective, lived experience of a resident is a perfect way to try and repattern old thoughts and stereotypes about the elderly.

STUDENT ACTION

Although Susan's planned learning was to brush up on her ambulating skills, she discovered a rich, unplanned learning experience as well. We are sure that you often have such unplanned learning experiences. Some of these experiences escape but a momentary notice. This exercise will give you an opportunity to bring those pieces of serendipity learning back into focus. Review yesterday and the past week. Think about clients/patients you have interacted with over this time. Use the following outline to write about several serendipitous learning experiences.

SERENDIPITOUS LEARNING EXPERIENCE 1

1. Describe enough about the serendipitous learning situation, including your feelings, to recreate the scene and your mood that set the stage for your learning.

2. What meaning did you give to the experience? What significance did it hold for you beyond the immediate care of this client?

SERENDIPITOUS LEARNING EXPERIENCE 2

1. Describe enough about the situation, including your feelings, to recreate the scene and your mood that set the stage for your learning.

2. What meaning did you give to the experience? What significance did it hold for you beyond the immediate care of this client?

SERENDIPITOUS LEARNING EXPERIENCE 3

1. Describe enough about the situation, including your feelings, to recreate the scene and your mood that set the stage for your learning.

2. What meaning did you give to the experience? What significance did it hold for you beyond the immediate care for this client?

NOTES ON USE

Student Use. The cases that you have just written about may be true "paradigm cases" for you. That is, cases which influence how you view other people or issues, what you see, and what you fail to see.

Instructor Use. Use your own examples of serendipitous learning to initiate a sharing of the students' experiences. You can collect these stories and form a booklet or newsletter to be passed on to other students. You need to collect and talk about your own paradigm cases to complete the circle of learning. Paraphrasing or summarizing other's comments, such as the class as a whole or a certain classmate, is an excellent way to identify paradigms and their attendant assumptions. Chubinski (1996) describes a critical thinking exercise for class: (1) a student is asked to summarize the class discussion up to a certain point as well as the dominant point of view taken by the class; (2) another student is asked to provide an alternative viewpoint; and (3) the class discusses how the alternative viewpoint challenges the assumptions of the original class perspective. This article contains other suggestions for developing critical thinking skills and reflection.

LEARNING TOOL 6.5

Listening to My Inner Dialogue

JOURNAL FOCUS

By staying in tune with your own internal dialogue while interacting with others in authority, such as your instructor, your own ability to learn from clinical experiences will increase and you may become more aware of personal thoughts and feelings that can impede effective listening and learning.

STUDENT WRITING

Think about yourself in previous interactions with others in authority. Reflect on the following situations and what your *inner dialogue or self-talk* might have been. Write down the inner dialogue for each, including your feelings and thoughts.

1. You are criticized for something that you did not do, but were supposed to do.

2. You are criticized for something that you did, but did not do well.

3. You are praised for something routine that you did well.

4. You are praised for something you did not so well at, but your attempt was appreciated.

POSITIVE STATEMENTS ABOUT ME

Remember, at the end of each journal entry you are to draw out from your reflections and journal writing positive statements you can make about yourself. Make each statement an "I" statement.

NOTES ON USE

Student Use.   This piece of learning can be applied to all situations to learn about yourself. By monitoring your thoughts and feelings, you can become more aware of your competence and correct course when thoughts get negative. Don't keep this to yourself—share your awareness with others and teach others to pay more attention to their self-talk.

Instructor Use.   This is a "teach by example" type of exercise. Use "I" statements to initiate a discussion about the self-talk that you have experienced in clinical situations. Encourage students to approach themselves with a sense of humor.

CHAPTER

7

Reviewing Your Competencies

JOURNAL THOUGHT

My patient talked to me — I mean really talked to me about family, many losses, and coping with those losses. My patient was very emotional during this time and I wondered if I had done something wrong.

NURSING STUDENT

PUTTING IT ALL TOGETHER: PREEVALUATION

Assessing your progress is an integral component of learning—as essential as planning, implementing, and evaluating client care. Just as you need to determine the quality of client care, you need to engage in a parallel process for yourself to determine the quality of your learning. Progress meetings are designed to highlight and review your developing competencies for nursing care. This form of feedback will occur many times throughout your nursing career. Although feedback is provided regularly in supervision from your instructor, there are usually two formal structured review or evaluation sessions during the clinical rotation.

Midterm and final evaluation interviews focus on progress. The review process is comprised of three elements. There are preevaluation activities, the evaluation interview itself, and postevaluation activities. Both you and your instructor engage in preevaluation meeting activities. Part of self-assessment, preparation activities include organizing and reviewing information about your knowledge, practice, and results to date. In the evaluation interview both you and your instructor will assess your progress and reach conclusions about whether you are "putting it all together" as you move from novice to informed learner along the continuum to becoming a professional nurse. Postevaluation activities focus on self-reflection and organizing yourself for improvement.

Assessing the Circle of Learning

Reviewing your competencies requires making decisions about *what* you have done during the clinical rotation, and *how you think* about what you have done. Assessing your learning requires you to pay attention to how well you are able to describe what you have been thinking about what you do, what you know, and what you've achieved. This is also called performance feedback. Feedback, is a form of communication to transmit information about the results of actions to the person who performed the actions—in this case information is communicated to you, the nursing student. Performance feedback is used to help students make modifications in nursing care; to increase the likelihood of continued growth; to help students recognize patterns that need improvement; and to give students positive indicators about evidence of growth in their thinking and ability to achieve appropriate nursing care.

The circle of learning strategies suggested throughout this book focus on thinking, doing, and knowing skills. Such information is derived from journal writing, paradigm cases, reading, observations, supervision, the practice portfolio, psychomotor lab, learning tools from this book, and other sources such as clients, peers, and collaterals or assignments. It is helpful to visualize the learning process as an ongoing feedback circle. Retention of information, application of theory, and integration of theory and practice is a circular process of learning that creates a continuous feedback source.

Nursing students need to appreciate that learning and progress is a highly individual process and each evaluation is thus individualized. Depending on your stage of learning, each student is also working at a different point along the learning continuum. The process of evaluation begins the moment you start your clinical rotation. Evaluative feedback continually comes from many sources—self and others, and from engaging in the learning tools suggested in this book—values exploration, knowledge building, critical thinking development, application enhancement, and journal writing. With these information sources in mind, the sample evaluation form in Appendix E can be used as a guide to prepare for your evaluation interview. Each nursing education program will have its own evaluation forms, but the core elements of accepted practice are consistent. Use the evaluation form that is specific to your practicum to identify examples of when you met expectations and how you would rate yourself. Remember, the review of competencies will focus on what you know, what you have been doing, and what the resulting outcomes are of your nursing care.

Reviewing What You Know

What do you know? You know a great deal, and since day one of the practicum you have been thinking critically about this. Information about what you know has been organized and compiled in various formats to record your accomplishments during this time (your practice portfolio). Reviewing (values exploration and critical thinking) what you know (knowledge building) and how that was demonstrated (application enhancement and journal writing) is important information to evaluate your competencies. Organizing and interpreting your thinking, doing, and your results will prepare you for the evaluation interview.

Reviewing what you know is a self-assessment feedback process that determines to what extent you are acquiring the necessary core elements and competencies of professional nursing practice. You will search all of your information sources for both your successes and setbacks. As noted earlier in this book (see Chapter 6), learning comes from what you do and what you understand about what you do. Learning comes from acting and responding to the feedback from your mistakes, your successes, and your understandings.

Discovering *all* of your strengths and concerns is not necessary and usually impossible. Remember, your instructors are experienced nurses who will offer their observations and feedback of your progress using the criteria developed by the nursing program. After all, that is their role as your instructor.

Reviewing What You Do

What did you do during the practicum? When evaluating your nursing practice and skills, start with where you began. Review the learning plan and goals you set for yourself. What did you do in your nursing role? What did you do in your practice and thinking to meet your learning needs? Be honest about your learning and progress as you review your information sources—your journal, paradigm cases, logs, records, and practice portfolio. What did you actually do? What did you hope to do? What explains any discrepancies? What did you do that was not planned? Were nursing interventions based on client circumstances and safety? Did your nursing care meet professional standards of care? Were you comfortable in providing the nursing care? Did you respond to diverse client needs by developing culturally competent or culturally sensitive nursing care?

Reviewing Your Results

What are the results of your individual and collective nursing care? The best way to review your results will be to review your successes, accomplishments, and setbacks. Review the narrative accounts from your journal entries, case records including your paradigm case, supervision, and the practice portfolio (see Chapter 6). The task is to "pull out" from these various sources *moments of learning* that illustrate progress, change, and results. You are constructing the information to create an integrated view of yourself—the nursing student and learner. Review these incidents and moments of learning with a comparative analysis of your written learning plan. What do you think about the results? Are you pleased? Are you concerned about some aspects of your development? If so, what areas raise questions for your development? Reflect on your learning goals, then identify opportunities from your nursing care that demonstrate the repetition or maintenance of skills and knowledge. Did you demonstrate the application of these skills to new situations? In other words, were you able to generalize your achievements or change across time and across assignments and tasks? Are positive patterns and competent skills repeated? Incorporating new learning repeatedly into nursing care practice demonstrates integration of learning and promotes improved performance. If you needed to unlearn certain patterns and skills did this also occur? Questions to ask yourself as you reflect on what you know, what you did, and your results include:

- What have I learned?
- What are my successes?
- What were my setbacks?
- What kind of a problem is there (if at all)?
- Where does the problem occur?
- When does the problem occur?
- What does it add up to?
- What do I need to do more of?

* What do I need to do differently?

    * How will I know when I achieve my goals?

Preparing for Constructive Feedback

Each day, there are many learning moments in the practicum when feedback is forthcoming. Therefore, by the time midterm evaluation arrives, there should be no surprises about your progress. Again, start thinking about the review of your competencies early in the practicum; in fact, if you keep the narrative accounts suggested in this book, your task will be easier. Narrative accounts of practice can convey whether you are developing competence and confidence in your nursing role, in your nursing practice, and in your critical thinking. As with all of your work, critical thinking is required in the preevaluation review.

    Evaluation feedback typically elicits a range of feelings, emotions, and even value conflicts for nursing students. Be sure to consider the type of constructive feedback you would give yourself, which can help you anticipate constructive feedback of your instructor during the evaluation interview. Constructive feedback will take the form of noting specific positive aspects of your performance and specific suggestions for improvement. Students often consider the suggestions for change and improvement as criticism. Critical comments should be avoided and balanced with suggestions and examples of progress. Remember your preferred learning approaches? Some learning styles of students focus only on grades and criticism. Students with these learning styles cannot see the "big picture" of their progress.

    Decide ahead of time how you handle constructive feedback. Do you focus on concerns? Is it hard to keep your feelings under control? Personalize and take responsibility for your feelings and reactions. Assess your style and determine what you need to do in advance to handle this communication. Some students like to ask for more details and examples or ask what solutions would solve a problem. You can keep a cool head by planning in advance. Steps include stopping, calming down, and thinking. Describe the problem and how you feel. Acknowledge the position for your instructor and raise questions about the observations. Request clarification, support your suggestions with evidence, and *compromise when appropriate*. If you can spot your setbacks and concerns in advance, and propose suggestions for improvement, then you are well on your way to handling feedback constructively.

⁖ THE EVALUATION INTERVIEW

The midterm evaluation interview occurs about midway through the practicum. The final evaluation interview is just that, an evaluation interview at the end of the rotation. These two assessment periods are designed to provide a more formal appraisal of your nursing abilities. Some nursing programs may require additional assessment times, and/ or some students may need additional assessment interviews. There are common processes in all of these interviews. The evaluation interview is a meeting where you and your instructor bring together all of the information about your accomplishments, and then consider and discuss the results. In some situations, the evaluation interview will include you and your instructor, as well as your preceptor.

The Process

All nursing students will feel anxiety or distress about the evaluation process itself. Some students will feel more stress than others. Some students may even believe that the evaluation process interferes with their ability to work effectively during clinical rotation. *Anxiety is normal.* Most students realize and welcome the knowledge building and benefits derived from this form of feedback even though it is stressful. Remind yourself that this is part of your learning. Evaluations will be a reality throughout your career. Evaluation forms part of nursing's ongoing professional development long after you leave your education program. There are benefits not only to you, but also to the profession and clients. Just as you evaluate client progress, your evaluation informs you about the potential ways you need to change, improve, or enhance performance. Evaluation is invaluable.

The Content

Both you and your instructor will arrive at the evaluation interview with the information you prepared in advance of the meeting. The content will focus on your competencies with examples from your practice. Various areas of practice competencies will be reviewed. You will have an opportunity to discuss the findings with your instructor. Areas of agreement will be balanced with concerns for improvement. Request clarification and information where appropriate, and balance talking and listening in a way that increases the likelihood of attaining an informed perspective about your performance.

A written evaluation is the result of this process. Your progress will be judged as satisfactory or unsatisfactory. Different programs will use different terminology about satisfactory progress—for example, you may receive a grade, a credit, or a pass or fail. This will vary from program to program, but in essence each program will look at whether your overall progress is satisfactory in various areas. The content of the evaluation interview provides you with information about your instructor's assessment of what you understand and what you do not; what you can do in your nursing care and what you cannot; which aspects of your nursing care are effective and which are not.

ASSESSING POSTEVALUATION OUTCOMES

Assessing postevaluation outcomes provides you with a chance to engage in critical thinking after the evaluation interview. In the quiet of your own space, you will need to reflect on the evaluation experience and to write about your reactions to the process in your journal. Reread the written report. Dialogue with yourself and listen to the response. As usual, you need to record your emerging strengths and speak to the positives. For areas of practice requiring improvement you will have to decide how to clarify concerns and problems and the options for resolving them. Do you have a representative picture of where you have been and where you are going in this journey toward becoming an informed learner? Your understanding and reactions to the evaluation will guide your next steps. Given your achievements, what do you need to do to move forward? This, of course, will depend on whether you received a satisfactory or unsatisfactory evaluation.

Strategies for assessing postevaluation outcomes include:

- Clearly identify conclusions and milestones.
- Avoid overstating your concerns or strengths.
- Create a chart or graph from the evaluation report to facilitate a visual analysis of your progress.
- Reflect on the explanations for the results.
- Always stress accuracy and honesty with yourself in reviewing your accounts of learning.

Notes

Satisfactory Progress

Congratulations if you received a satisfactory progress report. Your instructor probably indicated where you needed to continue doing more of the same, and where change or improvement is needed. You may have agreed in total or in part with the evaluation. What matters is that you still have time to improve your competencies. At this point your task is to revise your learning plan to continue to make progress. Specific suggestions may have been communicated to you about what areas you need to know or learn, and perhaps aspects of your thinking and doing you may need to unlearn. A satisfactory report does not mean that you can sit back and relax for the next half of the term. Your task is to keep journaling, keep your paradigm cases for future reexamination, and to keep thinking critically in order to continue growing and learning in the desired direction. Achieving change and maintaining desired behaviors, skills, and attitudes is just as important for the next phase of the clinical rotation. Becoming a caring nurse and providing nursing care are both developmental and socialization processes. A satisfactory evaluation is one step in the journey, albeit an important step.

Unsatisfactory Progress

Students who receive an unsatisfactory progress report at the evaluation interview usually have an idea that difficulties are present in their nursing care. Difficulties are often pointed out during direct supervision and in daily feedback during the course of the clinical rotation to help students make the necessary changes prior to the evaluation interview. Sometimes instructors feel that they have made it very clear that a student's performance is not up to par, but the student has not "heard" that message. Instructors do not give unsatisfactory ratings without prior warnings. If you have received information about your lack of progress and don't know how to improve, talk it over with your instructor and try to work out a plan for the specific learning. If you are really worried about your progress and are not sure if the feedback you are getting constitutes a warning, clarify that with your instructor. Don't wait for the evaluation interview. Some students worry needlessly because they have interpreted any constructive feedback as negative.

An unsatisfactory progress report is, of course, very disappointing and stressful. It is the persistence of difficulties and concerns that can result in an unsatisfactory review. What does a satisfactory progress report mean to you? What does an unsatisfactory progress report mean to you? A student's attitude toward learning can often warrant an unsatisfactory progress warning.

Becoming defensive in the face of a disappointing evaluation is not productive or desirable, but it is perhaps excusable. However, if you are habitually defensive, if you always respond to criticism with denial or anger, it will be impossible for your practicum instructor to teach you. If she cannot teach you, it will be impossible for you to achieve your minimum learning goals and objectives that are required for you to pass your practicum.

Your practicum instructor will always make allowances for a family crisis, an ailing automobile, or a life-threatening illness that keeps you away from the agency for a day or two. If the illness is really life-threatening, or if you have really suffered some personal disaster, arrangements may be made for you to make up the lost time, extend the practicum over a long period of time, or even withdraw from the practicum with and "incomplete." An "incomplete" means that you can finish the practicum at a later date after you have coped with your personal disaster.

If you habitually avoid certain situations, clients, or types of client problems and issues, offering flimsy excuses, if you are frequently late, or if you take two-hour lunch breaks or go home early, your practicum instructor will mention it to you. If you fail to mend your ways after repeated reminders, the result may very well be an "unsatisfactory" rating at your mid-term evaluation. (Thomlison et al., 1996, p. 211).

An unsatisfactory report may be a warning, suggesting that unless major changes in behavior and attitude are forthcoming a failing grade will be given. It may also mean that you cannot proceed further at this point, especially if safety is a major concern, or that you have failed and must withdraw from the clinical rotation. A program may or may not allow for an evaluation appeal. Some programs may provide the opportunity for you to repeat part or all of the clinical rotation. An unsatisfactory report may mean that you cannot proceed and have to withdraw from the nursing program. It may even mean you are not suitable to nursing. If this is the case, it can indeed be a very distressful time for you. Some common difficulties resulting in an unsatisfactory progress review include:

- Unsafe practice such as medication errors and lack of client care and attention, e.g., failing to check patient identification
- Unprofessional, unethical, or unsafe conduct
- Insufficient knowledge base (e.g., pathophysiology, medications), serious problems in applying information to direct situations
- Inability to recognize difficulties and make changes
- Unprofessional behavior and attitude
- Failure to seek help as needed

If you believe that you have been evaluated unfairly, you usually have a right to appeal the decision. This first step though is always to try to work it through with your instructor. If you and your instructor cannot reach a satisfactory agreement, and you still believe the decision is unfair, it is appropriate to ask to meet with the practicum coordinator. Most nursing programs have formal procedures for appeal. There will be a deadline for submitting an appeal, but there is always time to think over what your instructor has said, the concerns that have been presented, and the supporting evidence. It is understandable to feel upset and even a bit defensive. But be honest with yourself. Repeating a course, if that is one of your options, can be beneficial in the long run. Realizing that you need to make some changes in your behavior is sobering, but not an endpoint.

Suitability to Nursing.   Perhaps you are not suited to the profession of nursing. You may have reached this conclusion from your self-assessment or from talking with your instructor. The reasons may not be at all clear to you, or you may have discovered the personal and academic qualities needed for nursing are not a good fit with you. Some students are not ready for professional practice. You may be experiencing personal and life stressors, in which case you are not emotionally or psychologically available to help others and may place them at risk of harm. Some students may have engaged in unethical or unacceptable practices. There are many reasons a student may not be suitable and it is the instructor's function to communicate this. Although this may be difficult to face, it can also be an opportunity for further learning. As discussed in other parts of this book, some of the most meaningful learning emerges from the failures and setbacks. While it may not be evident to you now, it is important to realize that this learning can often set you on a pathway where you are more suited and successful. When you let your strengths take you in other directions, this "setback" can result in future successes. Remember that the evaluation interview is not an end in itself, but a way for you and your instructor to gain clarity about your directions.

LEARNING FOR IMPROVEMENT

In nursing, self-assessment and self-improvement are important qualities for learning. Knowing how to capitalize on success, when to ask for help, and positively managing constructive feedback are all paramount to your ongoing development. Successful students acknowledge when they do not know a procedure or medication, they concede the difference between an honest mistake and careless practice. Learning is an active strategy and is a matter of building on existing knowledge and thinking skills. Research indicates that integration is more likely to occur when information is repeated. Consistency in preparation for practice is key. Review your narrative accounts of practice and your reactions several times as you develop your strategies for ongoing learning.

Your Reactions

Nursing students typically have mixed reactions to the evaluation interview. You may not agree with the feedback from your instructor and you may be filled with doubts and questions about developing abilities. Students often focus on concerns while forgetting the positive feedback from the evaluation. Dwelling on the negatives or concerns, such as blaming others for your lack of progress, can be self-handicapping. Enhancing and maintaining your critical thinking skills will help you view any uncertainties and setbacks as learning opportunities leading to improvement.

Accountability and Responsibility

Reviewing your competencies has implications apart from your learning needs. Developing competencies for nursing practice is also about accountability and responsibility. You are accountable to yourself, to the nursing profession, to your clients, to the health-care organization in which your work, and to other stakeholder systems, such as funders, or other collateral agencies. In fact, accountability and responsibility for the provision of safe, quality services have long been part of nursing values and ethics. There are common elements pertaining to accountable and responsible practice among the international, American, and Canadian nursing codes of ethics (see Appendixes A, B, and C). All three codes refer to the professional obligation of nurses to ensure and safeguard the client and the public. The incompetent, unethical, or illegal practice by any person is not tolerated. It is the responsibility of each individual to provide competent and ethical nursing care, as well as contribute to advancing knowledge building to meet the health needs of the public. Ongoing evaluation is, therefore, considered as an essential aspect of ethical, safe, and accountable nursing care.

Reexamining Your Thinking

Now that you are less stressed and less emotional, it is time to return to journal writing. Reexamine your thinking for future directions.

1. Reviewing your thinking assists you in identifying and assessing the impact of practice tasks and actions.

2. Reviewing your thinking provides evidence of improvement and is instrumental in helping you maintain an effective motivation level and commitment to learning.

3. Reviewing your thinking will provide you with objective information to report at supervision.

4. Consistent use of journaling and writing in the practice portfolio promotes a more objective, systematic approach to growth and development.

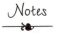

5. Each journal entry needs at least one positive statement about your abilities or strengths.

6. Reviewing your narrative accounts helps you identify themes, patterns, and accomplishments.

   Reviewing your thinking helps you feel more confident to approach related learning issues in the future.

Reexamining Your Doing

Reexamining your achievements helps you to integrate them into the daily functions of nursing care for maximum learning. This is best accomplished throughout the clinical rotation by emphasizing and practicing learned skills and behaviors in a variety of situations and across different examples.

Reaching Conclusions

What conclusions have you reached?

- One of the most important ways of learning to move forward now is to change your focus from *what* you are thinking to *how* you are thinking.

- The context of critical thinking for nursing care improves assessment, planning, and interventions.

- Feedback in the form of evaluation is the planned opportunity to enhance your thinking, doing, and practice skills, and continue to learn. It is a necessary part of leaning to be a professional. It is an opportunity to discuss and understand the impact of nursing care dynamics and how these elements affect responses of nurses.

SUMMARY

Preevaluation, the evaluation interview, and postevaluation activities are part of a continuous feedback process to learning. These activities involve the careful preparation and attention to your narrative accounts and activities.

- Review what you know.
- Review what you did.
- Decide where you need to go.

Evaluation must form a part of routine and sound nursing care. Evaluation promotes self-assessment and self-improvement focused on what you know, what you have been doing, and what the results are for developing competencies.

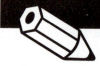

LEARNING TOOL 7.1

Self-Evaluation

LEARNING FOCUS: Values Exploration

Dealing with evaluation, hopefully constructive evaluation, requires learned skills and preparation. No one enjoys being evaluated, but you can learn to deal effectively with evaluation so that you can learn from the experience. Preparing well for your evaluation will help you to reduce anxiety and to know yourself better.

STUDENT ACTION

This exercise pulls together many pieces of your learning.

1. Make a list of practice pieces that you do well.

    Practice Pieces I Do Well

2. Now make a list of practice pieces that you could have done differently or skills in which you need to improve your performance.

    Correcting Course

NOTES ON USE

Student Use.   This exercise is a preparation for your evaluation interview. To prepare, you will need to review many sources of information. For example, review course outlines for the knowledge, attitudes, and skills that are expected for each course. Check any feedback situations that you have recorded in your journal or in other ways throughout the practicum. Remember that you have to pay attention to what you know and what you can do. Use some way of measuring your level of performance. You can rate yourself from 1 to 10, but be sure you are able to describe what your performance at a certain level looks like. It is best to anchor your measurements by defining performance at levels 1, 5, and 10 on your scale. That way you can compare your "7" rating as about halfway between how you defined level 5 and level 10. An alternative performance measure is the Taxonomy of Psychomotor Behavior in Chapter 3.

Instructor Use.   Self-evaluation can be quite scary for students. They often feel ill prepared to assess their own performance. Preparing for an evaluation interview is an excellent way to work on the issues of subjective feelings and perceptions and collecting more objective evidence for assessing performance and knowledge. You can teach students how to develop an anchored self-rating scale by looking at the graduated levels of knowledge or performance and affixing a numerical rating to these levels. To help students keep their performance in perspective, use examples where students span the spectrum of skill or knowledge proficiency. Students can practice breaking things down into skill levels by working in pairs and using common skills such as taking a shower or bath. This helps students learn to develop anchored scales to assess client/patient skill levels as well.

LEARNING TOOL 7.2

Making Feedback Constructive

LEARNING FOCUS: Knowledge Building

Preevaluation planning for handling the emotions elicited during evaluation interviews can be very helpful in experiencing the feedback as constructive. Learning from the feedback is the purpose of evaluation.

STUDENT ACTION

Here are some strategies for reframing feedback that will help you to increase the benefit of constructive feedback. For each strategy, write how using the strategy will help you when you encounter critical feedback in your clinical experiences.

1. Keep in mind what is at stake—take the long view. Put criticism into the perspective of your ultimate goal.

2. Don't throw the baby out with the bathwater. The delivery of the criticism may need improvement, but look beyond that to the message.

3. Write down a way that you have developed to reframe criticism that helps you deal with the situation and learn from it.

Anticipate and decide ahead of time how you will handle critical feedback. Answering the following questions will help you make a preevaluation interview plan.

1. Do you tend to focus on concerns and dismiss the positives? How will you adopt a more balanced approach in this interview?

2. Is it hard for you to keep your feeling intensity under control? What are the telltale signs that feeling intensity is rising? For example, do your cheeks or neck get red? What corrective actions could you use to minimize these signs? For example, wear a turtleneck or take notes to help you stay focused on what is being said rather than how you are feeling.

3. Do you take responsibility for your feelings or are you into blaming—he/she made me feel that? What maxim could you recall to encourage yourself to take responsibility for your own feelings?

4. Assess your style and determine what you need to do in advance to handle this type of communication. If you were to rehearse potential evaluation scenarios with someone, what areas would you practice?

5. Keep a cool head—stop, calm down, and think! What strategies could you do to remember this? Maybe a maxim would help.

NOTES ON USE

Student Use.   Remember your preferred learning approach when you do this exercise and see how they are linked. Your preparation will probably be more extensive than is needed, but it will help you to feel more emotionally ready to handle the evaluation interview. Your knowledge and performance will be assessed by clients or family members as well as other professionals throughout your nursing experience. Any preparing you do for this formal evaluation can be applied to other situations in the clinical setting and in life.

Instructor Use.   Provide the students with practice in dealing with critical comments. Collect a number of situations from the practicum where students have received or witnessed critical comments from patients/clients, family, or other professionals. Have the students work in triads with each scenario: one student is the person making the critical comment; one student is the recipient of the comments; and the third student is a coach to encourage the recipient to use strategies to handle the situation. Students can practice strategies such as requesting clarification of specific examples, rephrasing critical comments to ensure that others understand what they heard, or asking for suggestions to resolving problems. Triads should report back to the class the strategies that were effective in this situation for this student. Remind students that they can use these effective strategies for handling any situation where they feel criticized.

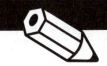

LEARNING TOOL 7.3

Strengths and Concerns

LEARNING FOCUS: Critical Thinking Development

You have been collecting information from various sources to help you decide about your learning outcomes, strengths, and concerns. Guidelines for thinking critically about the explanations of your strengths and concerns may be clustered into at least three areas: changes in attitude, changes in skills, and changes in behavior.

STUDENT ACTION

Utilize a variety of sources (e.g., pragmatic, narrative, and objective) for specific evidence of changes in each of the following categories of learning—circumstances, attitude, skills, and behavior). A *narrative source* might be from your journal where you identify themes and patterns repeated in practice and thinking. *Objective sources* might be scores from assignments and comments from expert nurses who viewed your work. These should be in your practice portfolio for easy access. *Pragmatic evidence* can be found in the increased speed with which you are able to perform nursing procedures due to changes in your skill and confidence levels. Under each of the following categories, list at least one expected attitude, skill, or behavior; the type of evidence (pragmatic, etc.); a brief description of the evidence and/or counterevidence; and the conclusions you might draw from the evidence (i.e., your strengths or concerns).

CHANGES IN ATTITUDE

1. Attitude (e.g., increased self-awareness, self-confidence, help-seeking):

2. Evidence Type (Specify type(s) of evidence you have for this attitude—narrative, objective and/or pragmatic):

3. Evidence/Counterevidence (e.g., feedback from instructor after observing me with a patient):

4. Conclusions (Describe your strengths and/or concerns regarding how you have changed in this attitude.):

CHANGES IN SKILLS

1. Skill (e.g., increased psychomotor skills, communication skills):

2. Evidence Type (Specify the type(s) of evidence you have for this skill—narrative, objective and/or pragmatic):

3. Evidence/Counterevidence:

4. Conclusions (Describe your strengths and/or concerns regarding how you have changed in this skill.):

CHANGES IN BEHAVIOR OR DOING

1. Attitude (e.g., increased knowledge and critical thinking skills, a sense of humor):

2. Evidence Type (Specify the type(s) of evidence you have for this behavior—narrative, objective and/or pragmatic):

3. Evidence/Counterevidence:

4. Conclusions (Describe your strengths and/or concerns regarding how you have changed in this behavior.):

Now reexamine your sources or types of evidence.

1. Have you been relying on one type of evidence or do you have a fair mix?

2. What type of evidence occurs most frequently?

3. Are some types of evidence more suited to specific kinds of strengths or concerns?

4. How do you think the reliance on types of evidence is related to your preferred learning style?

NOTES ON USE

Student Use.   This exercise gives you an opportunity to classify the type of evidence you are drawing upon, as well as to consider what conclusion the evidence supports. These are important skills not only for your own performance but in assessing clients/patients as well. You can enrich this exercise in several ways. First, you can list a number of attitudes, skills, and behaviors expected of you so far in this practicum and complete the four steps for each of these rather than just one. Also, you can write about times when you had to assess the attitudes, skills and/or behavior of clients, and the sources of evidence you used or could have used to reach your conclusions.

Instructor Use.   Ask students to bring their completed assignments to class. Choose which section (i.e., attitudes, skills, or behavior) is least threatening for students to begin their sharing. Have students each share the one attitude, skill, or behavior they chose to highlight. Create a master list of these skills, attitudes, and behaviors. Add to the list things that have not been mentioned by any student. Discuss with students any patterns or themes in the skills, attitudes, and behaviors they chose.

LEARNING TOOL 7.4

Postevaluation Care Plan

LEARNING FOCUS: Application Enhancement

Throughout your nursing education, care planning will hold a dominant place in your learning. After the stress of an evaluation, it is time to use those skills on yourself and with classmates.

STUDENT ACTION

This time you are the case example. Recall the nursing process: assessment, planning, implementing, and evaluating.

1. Review your records! Based on past experiences with evaluation situations, what are your hunches as to your emotional state prior to and after the evaluation interview?

2. What conclusions can you make about your physical, emotional, and social needs following the evaluation? Separate immediate and short-term needs.

3. Write down how to help yourself respond to your postevaluation condition. Which aspects of your needs take priority? What are your physical, emotional, and social goals?

4. What specific activities would help you carry out these goals? Remember to specify what you would do, and how, when, where, and why you would do it.

NOTES ON USE

Student Use.   Self-care is your responsibility. Knowing yourself and your needs is important in any situation but especially so in emotionally charged situations like evaluations. Each person is different in what they need and how best to fill those needs after an evaluation. Some people have high social needs, while others need a period of quiet before they can celebrate with others. Planning is helpful but do not be a slave to the plan. Be as flexible and as adaptive as you would be with a client. It's okay for you to change your mind. Use the feedback you get from the physical, emotional, and spiritual aspects of yourself to gauge what modifications you need to make to your plan.

Instructor Use.   As outlined in this exercise, the nursing process can be applied to personal situations. You can provide other opportunities to reinforce the principles of this process by using it in everyday life to approach everyday problems or situations. This will help students become familiar with applying the process to specific situations.

LEARNING TOOL 7.5

The Review Process

JOURNAL FOCUS

Reflecting on the evaluation process takes time, but it is time well spent. You want to get the most out of all your learning and reflecting will tease out bits of learning that you did not know were there.

STUDENT ACTION

The first set of questions will help you to collect and review journal writings over several months as part of the preevaluation process. The second set of questions will help you to create a journal reflection postevaluation.

PREEVALUATION REVIEW

1. What have I learned?

2. What are my successes?

3. What were my setbacks?

4. What kind of problem(s) have I encountered (if at all)?

5. Where and when do the problem(s) occur? Is there a pattern?

6. What does it add up to?

7. What do I need to do more of?

8. What do I need to do differently?

9. How will I know when I achieve my goals?

POSTEVALUATION REVIEW

1. Compare your assessment of your strengths and your concerns to the strengths and concerns raised by your instructor. How are they similar and dissimilar?

2. Did you over- or underestimate your knowing, doing, or thinking in any area(s)? What were they?

3. How do you make sense of this?

4. Is this similar to other evaluations? Is there a pattern?

5. What can you take forward for the next evaluation? Remember the maxims—do more of the same if it is working well and try another way if it is not!

POSITIVE STATEMENTS ABOUT ME

Remember, at the end of each journal entry you are to draw out from your reflections and journal writing positive statements you can make about yourself. Make each statement an "I" statement.

NOTES ON USE

Student Use.   Preevaluation, the evaluation interview, and postevaluation are part of a continuous feedback process to your learning. Evaluation must form part of your routine and sound nursing care. The evaluation process promotes self-assessment and self-improvement. This process may be relevant for some of the clients with whom you work as well. For example, learning to live with diabetes is a complex and ongoing process. How might you offer feedback to clients on their learning about their own health and illness?

Instructor Use.   Coaching students to take an increasingly active role in self-evaluation is a challenging but important process. The value of this learning tool is its emphasis on helping students look for their own patterns over time. To some students this may be an easy process; to others it may be more difficult. You might want to ask students to hand in this exercise and then go over it with them individually.

PART FOUR

Transition Tools

Learning as a Journey

JOURNAL THOUGHT

I heard of the challenges of caring for my patient from some of the other students. The child was very independent and could become quite demanding and hysterical. I used the concept of industry versus inferiority to give her a sense of control. My patient was quite nervous and anxious that I might hurt her, so I suggested that she could do it while I supervised. In a way, I put her in the teacher position. I gave my patient gloves and assisted her while at the same time talking to her about preventing infection. This was amazing. She did an excellent job and not one cry of pain. She even suggested to her roommate that she try to do her pin site herself.

One example was with her pin site care.

NURSING STUDENT

Matters related directly or indirectly to the practicum deserve considerably more space than provided here. The goal of this book is to guide you through the practicum phases from beginning to end, in an effort to help you make discoveries about yourself and the joy of nursing. Based on the discoveries and experiences of your practica, it is hoped that you are more encouraged and more open to learning and regularly seeking consultation, supervision, and critical thinking. The suggestions presented here are intended to highlight the key issues as you attempt to put all of the elements of critical thinking into perspective. Regardless of experience, nursing students report that clinical rotations are never forgotten and hold a special place in their memories.

Because of the special meaning clinical rotations hold for students, there are mixed emotions when it comes time to leave. You just started to feel as if you knew your way around the setting; you just started to become used to the routine, you remember names and faces now; and you have become attached to clients. However, it is time to make the transition to your next challenge. Before you leave, there are some matters requiring attention.

PREPARING TO LEAVE

Preparing to leave your client, instructor, and practicum typically elicits a range of feelings, emotions, and conflicts for students. When you started the practicum, the end probably didn't seem like one of those issues you needed to pay attention to, but you actually can be prepared for termination. Preparing for leaving or ending is focused on transitions to new experiences and support systems.

Leaving Clients

In reality, you start to prepare for leaving your clients, instructor, and practicum the day you start. Each contact or task you engage in has a beginning and ending. Each contact in a sense has a "good-bye" and is filled with emotion. As you bring your contact with your client to a close, it is helpful to review what you have accomplished and how the client is going to continue to receive help. In some cases, this means introductions to a new nurse or helper, or a transfer to another setting for the client. It is helpful to remind clients shortly before your departure that you are leaving. Clients will also have feelings about leaving you and need to prepare for separation as well. If possible, it is nice to introduce the client to the new person who will be taking over your responsibilities. Introductions smooth the transition for clients.

Leaving Your Instructor

The final evaluation interview will signal the formal termination with your practicum instructor. Regardless of your relationship with and feelings about your instructor, it is important and necessary for the two of you to sit down and review the process of that relationship. What was helpful, great, or wonderful? What else could have been done to assist in your learning? In the same way your instructor provided feedback to you, it is helpful when students provide feedback to instructors about teaching style and teaching activities. Putting closure to your relationship with your instructor helps both of you address your feelings and emotions in a positive way. If there are any unfinished matters or issues that were never discussed, try to talk about them now and resolve them. The focus is not necessarily about changing opinions or positions. It may simply be a matter of agreeing to disagree; in fact, some issues can be left at that as a form of resolution. If you have constructive criticism to provide about your issues, give recommendations for how the situation might be changed or improved. Balance concerns with positives. What is important is that you reach an amicable position so that both of you can put it behind and move forward. This is important to your ongoing development and for a transparent communication style. As well, your instructor may be called upon to write you a future recommendation. In any case, she or he is a "colleague" in the same profession and you never know when your paths may cross in the future. The unwritten protocol is to thank your instructor as part of the ritual associated with leaving and ending. This can take the form of a card, personal comments, lunch, or other symbol of recognition of thanks.

Leaving the Setting

Preparing to leave the setting also needs to be handled appropriately. People in the setting have provided help and it is important to communicate your appreciation to them and what their support meant to your learning. Did you feel accepted? Was the staff approachable? Saying good-bye to various people in the setting does not necessarily mean a permanent parting. You may find yourself working with someone from the setting, or interacting with people and this setting in other contexts in the future. Reviewing your reactions and feelings about the setting is an important activity in your deliberations of future opportunities for work and learning. Students often express their thanks to others in the setting through a small token of appreciation—a flower, card, book, or chocolates.

Transitions and Continuity

Rituals are important and useful in transitions as a formal way to reduce anxiety about change and to manage continuity as you move forward. Transitions are a time to affirm identity and recognize the subjective aspects of our experiences. Transitions also are a form of celebration and preparation for the next stages along the continuum from novice to informed learner. As you begin the transition from leaving the practicum it is necessary to link what you know, what you have been doing, and what you learned to the patterns, themes, and stages of your learning and to the anticipated transitions.

There are many ways to celebrate your leaving and transition to new opportunities and challenges. Examine the rituals and ceremonies you engage in at times of leaving and ending in other parts of your life. In many respects, these are personal and must fit the purpose of the situation. You may wish to construct your own ritual and ceremony for leaving each practicum.

❧ LESSONS LEARNED

Transitions are processes, not events. Therefore, it is important to use your critical thinking skills once again. What are the lessons you've learned—from your journal writing, the learning tools, your paradigm cases, and from others? What are the discoveries and joys of learning in practicum? Ending should be a time for adding up what you've learned. Learning is never finished, you will leave with new ideas as an agenda for future issues. This is a time for you to identify your future learning agenda. Write these thoughts down in your journal.

Discoveries

Reflect on some of the influences and learning from your supervision experiences, clients, colleagues, and nursing processes. These experiences have added to your development and learning in countless ways; hopefully, only a few are viewed as less than ideal. Less positive experiences certainly will make you understand the influence a supervisor has on one's professional work and self-understanding. The most important discovery you can make is that you can be both a vulnerable learner and a competent nursing student at the same time. You have learned about nursing care, the learning/teaching styles of yourself and instructor, and the context of learning. You have also been a learner in differing capacities. These learning opportunities will prove influential in endless ways as you handle the many transitions and challenges ahead.

Perhaps you also discovered that you now view your instructor or preceptor in a different light than on your initial meeting—as more of an outstanding role model, mentor, coach, or colleague. Please say *thank you* to the individuals in your practicum who communicated encouragement and who demonstrated respect and trust in you. Send a card or write a note of your recognition or gratitude. Although your instructor and preceptor will not be expecting you to do this, it is especially appreciated when students take the time to communicate their thanks. There may be other individuals in the practicum who also stand out in your mind, who were helpful, friendly, or who were just "there for you." Whether you leave a letter of thanks, some type of gesture is in order.

Novice to Informed Learner to Expert—Eventually

This section could also have been called "if my friends could see me now . . . they wouldn't believe it . . ." Do you remember what you were thinking when you started the practicum? It is helpful to go back to those first days you wrote in your journal and consider the thoughts, feelings, and experiences you noted. What is different now? What made the differences? This is a good time to list your paradigm cases and how those situations affected your thinking, doing, and behavior. What role did supervision contribute to learning nursing care? Moving from novice to informed learner, and eventually to expert, is a decision to accept and seek ongoing supervision and self-appraisal as an essential part of learning throughout your professional career.

🕮 LEARNING AS A JOURNEY

It is important to also understand that the work of becoming an informed learner will continue after this clinical rotation ends. You will have unanswered questions. While you can handle yourself more effectively than at the beginning, you will not have nursing all figured out. Part of what you need to live with is the uncertainties.

Recognizing Uncertainties

Resist the temptation to feel as if you must tie up all the loose ends. Instead create an inventory for future work on your concerns. Note them in your journal. Acknowledging your strengths and evolving concerns is more helpful. It is not unusual to feel as if you are not ready to move on. In fact, your instructor may think you could benefit from more time in the clinical rotation. This is normal and does not to take away from what you know. Practice does make you more perfect. There will be plenty of time for that. The message here is to identify those areas you have learned as well as those areas where you need to focus attention on. Remember that the skills you develop are transferable to other situations.

Maintaining Skills

A new skill does not become part of your nursing repertoire of competencies until it is repeated. Skills need to be practiced and generalized to many other contexts. Therefore, review the inventory of skills from your practice portfolio and journal. Note these skills in a special part of your journal and practice portfolio so that you can build on them for your next practicum or place of work. The more you do the better you will stand out among your peers and the more competent your nursing skills will become.

Stress and Coping

Coping and caring are important aspects of learning to be a nurse. Although stress is a normal part of everyday life, as a nursing student stress can change you from a caring individual to an apathetic person if you do not address it. Regardless of whether the stressors come from your personal or student life, excessive or ongoing stress is the result of ineffective coping strategies. Learning to reduce stress is the key to preventing burnout, and there are numerous books about this topic. Self-care is probably the single most important strategy you can focus on to prevent burnout. Sleeping problems are generally the first signs of stress in your life, but there are others. Some of the signs of stress and ineffective coping strategies are:

- inability to sleep restfully;
- feeling disillusioned with nursing;
- frequently feeling tired or calling in sick;
- unable to concentrate or solve problems;
- feeling overwhelmed;
- working below your potential;
- avoiding clients or work; and
- feeling alone or that no one understands your needs.

If you identify problems with more than three of the items on this checklist, you need to examine your self-care strategies. Patient care suffers when self-care is neglected.

Self-Care

A nursing student's capacity for client care expands with self-care. You can draw on this understanding with self-awareness. Discover or tune in to your own feelings and issues as you struggle to find a balance between work and personal life. Understanding your own life and issues, as well as personal crises, can teach you a great deal about your clients' struggles and issues. Tuning in to the common ground and struggles of individuals can make you better prepared and more sensitive to the needs of your clients. Awareness develops self-responsibility.

Getting in touch with your thoughts and feelings is self-care. Your sense of well-being starts with finding time for you, getting a good night's sleep, and finding ways to relax. "Running on empty" is a sure sign of a lifestyle in the process of a meltdown. Read your body's signals and look for the hassles contributing to the stress and ineffective coping. Self-care means finding a balance and feeling spiritually centered. Listen to your inner self and be clear about your values. Listen to your body and "nurse" it back to a balanced state. Rest, proper nutrition, exercise, and some fun are in order. Assess what you do for entertainment during "down-time." Changes in these areas will result in more effective coping responses to stressors. If you find this doesn't change, talk to your instructor, seek professional guidance, or locate other sources of support rituals.

Linking and Leaving

Students often feel they need more time in a clinical rotation. This is true for additional practica. Learning is just beginning when you are introduced to a new practicum; you are always readjusting. You are readjusting to the situation you are leaving and readjusting to the situation you are about to start. Skills you developed in dealing with the clients in the clinical rotation are transferable to other settings. Linking skills and process from past learning to new learning is a way of investing and building on the knowledge structure. Draw on the tools and strategies discussed in this book. Open up the toolbox and look in to see the supports needed for transitions to new experiences. You will need to tune in to identify connections between clients and situations. The process and content of one client nursing experience will help you learn what is needed in the new client assignment.

Notes

LOOKING BACK TO LOOK AHEAD

Looking back helps us to look ahead. What lessons did you learn about yourself, the profession, or those with whom you interacted? Some of the learning can be summarized as:

- Recognize the limits of your ability.
- Understand that setbacks are opportunities for learning.
- Accept that supervision is a necessity.
- Prevent job stress.
- Enhance and maintain the values, knowledge, and skills of a professional.
- Realize that the quality of becoming rather than being captures the meaning of "professional or expert."
- Develop a culture of thoughtfulness in your setting.

Critical thinking is not always a comfortable experience. Take the steps for critical discussion. Both activities will better serve clients.

Roads Taken and Not Taken

You may have felt that you did not receive all of the experiences you hoped for during the clinical rotation, or you may have had experiences about which you had no choice. All of these experiences contribute to the frustrations and accomplishments of learning a special kind of work. The people and experiences you are dealing with are complex. As you travel down one road you will encounter new crossroads. Choices may be difficult at times, but choosing a pathway now does not mean you can never go down that road in the future. This is our way of saying although you really want to spend extra time in pediatrics, the community school assignment may turn out great and prove to be a valuable learning experience in the area of prevention services. Maybe you can view pediatrics more broadly than you initially thought. Roads taken and not taken can always be revisited.

Dialogue with Yourself

Finally, we hope that the dialogue you start with yourself will continue over your lifetime. Talking with yourself and listening to yourself in a continuous learning circle will result in acquiring that special recognition of expert.

As an expert nurse it is our sincere hope that someday you will have the opportunity to work with students who make all of this worthwhile. You do not have to be perfect to help or teach, and at times you may wonder if it is all worth it. As you take care of others, take care of yourself and always reflect on what has passed in order to keep the future in perspective.

SUMMARY

Learning as a journey is a process of change. Helen Harris Perlman (1989), a well-known social work educator, eloquently speaks to this journey when she states:

If looking back represents a reluctance to leave the known for the unknown, if it expresses a fear of present prospects, if it is a temptation to escape the here-and-now reality and thus becomes a deterrent to looking ahead with courage, it is to be deplored. If, however, it is a way of gaining perspective, a means by which we may recognize and thus avoid earlier errors of judgement and action, or if, in reverse, it is a means by which to identify and preserve what is still to be developed further, if, in short, we look to the past as a way of seeing more clearly and penetratingly its meanings, and uses for our immediate present and near-future, then it may serve us well. So my malaise is temporarily put to rest, and I look back in order to see ahead. (Perlman, 1989, pp.1–2).

LEARNING TOOL 8.1

Making and Marking Endings

LEARNING FOCUS: Values Exploration

Creating and using traditions or rituals associated with leaving or leave-taking are an important part of life as a nursing student. Throughout your education and practice as a nurse you will have to say many good-byes. Good-byes, endings, and transitions to new opportunities are indeed part of the very fabric of the nursing profession. This exercise will give you an opportunity to examine some of the rituals and ceremonies you engage in at times of leaving and ending.

STUDENT ACTION

Remember, the ways of marking transitions or endings are personal and must fit the purpose of the situation. With that in mind, reflect upon your past experiences with endings and complete the following.

1. Many of the endings that you will encounter as a nursing student are with clients/patients. What has been the most memorable good-bye with a client/patient? What made it so memorable? What did you contribute or what part did you play in the ending?

2. Consider the staff in your clinical practicum and how did you or would you like to say good-bye to these people. Are there traditional ways in your program for this? How can you make them personal?

3. What would be your way of marking the end of this clinical rotation and celebrating the growth you have experienced? What have you done in the past and how could you build upon that tradition?

NOTES ON USE

Student Use.   During your nursing program, you will be part of many different groups. Pay attention to how endings happen and to how you can shape those endings in ways that are meaningful to you.

Instructor Use.   You will need to decide how you want the class to say good-bye and how you want to express yourself to them. Do you have a traditional way of ending your work with students?

LEARNING TOOL 8.2

Constructing a Practice Profile

LEARNING FOCUS: Knowledge Building

This exercise will give you the opportunity to create or add to your practice profile for future clinical experiences. This clinical experience may be choosing a future practicum placement or applying for a nursing position. It will be important for you to gather together some specific ideas and information about yourself that may be relevant to selecting a particular clinical experience. This information should be kept in your practice portfolio for future reference and updating.

STUDENT ACTION

Fill in or check descriptors that most clearly represent your personal style, interests, and experiences.

PERSONAL ATTRIBUTES

Describe your major personality characteristics, such as passive, anxious, questioning, curious, or flexible.

List the top four character assets that you consider will stand you in good stead as a nurse.

1.

2.

3.

4.

List the three areas that you need to improve to become an effective nurse.

1.

2.

3.

Use a colored pen to mark the point where you see yourself in these characteristics of personal style. Now, use another color to mark the point where you would like to be in the future.

Frequent _____ Seldom

Use of Humor

Cautious _____ Risking
                                   Risk Taking

Distant _____ Intimate
                                  Relationships

Active _____ Reactive
                                 Taking Initiative

Quiet _____ Vivacious
                                   Temperament

CHARACTERISTICS OF THINKING

Place a mark at the point where you see yourself in these characteristics of cognitive style.

High _____ Low
                               Degree of Structure

Audio _____ Visual
                               Learning Method

Deductive _____ Inductive
                               Learning Approach

LIFE EXPERIENCES AND FUTURE NURSING GOALS

Describe your preference for working with a particular client/patient group based on significant past or present experiences. Describe the experiences that have formed your preferences.

Describe your preferences for avoiding work with a particular client/patient group based on significant past or present experiences. Describe the experiences that have formed your preferences.

LEARNING TOOL 8.2 continued

LONG-TERM CAREER PLANS

What experiences will be most useful in helping your career possibilities in the future?

PREVIOUS PROFESSIONAL EXPERIENCE

List any previous professional or volunteer experiences you have had.

COURSE WORK AND SKILLS TRAINING

List all classes and training that you have taken—certain courses may be specifically relevant to future clinical experiences.

LONG-TERM CAREER PLANS

What clinical rotation experiences will be most useful in helping your career possibilities in the future?

CLINICAL SETTINGS

Which clinical settings would best match your abilities and interests at this time? Indicate any course work or experience you have that relates to these clinical settings.

NURSING SPECIALIZATIONS OF INTEREST

What areas of nursing are you most interested in working in at this point in your nursing education? Outline any prior courses, training, or experience you have had in the areas of most interest (e.g., adult health and illness; child health; community health; critical care; family/newborn; international/out-of-region; mental health; rural; senior health).

LEARNING TOOL 8.2 continued

INTEGRATING THEORY AND PRACTICE

What theoretical orientation or treatment approach is most interesting to you at present? From course work and readings, how is your preferred approach utilized in your area of interest?

LEARNING OPPORTUNITIES

What type of learning opportunities do you hope to have in future clinical practicums? What level of involvement and responsibility would you prefer?

INSTRUCTOR STYLE AND PERSONALITY

What are the personal qualities of an instructor with whom you think you would work best? What personal styles might challenge you, yet be helpful in your learning?

LIMITATIONS

List any concerns you might have about the limits of your abilities or knowledge. Identify any concerns or questions you have about your personal safety or risks related to clinical rotation placements.

NOTES ON USE

Student Use.   You are in the midst of exciting professional development as a nurse. In answering these questions remember there are no right or wrong responses. Place this in your practice portfolio for further reference. Review this profile as you complete other clinical experiences. See where you are on your pathway of learning to be a nurse.

Instructor Use.   As an instructor you will have many opportunities for sharing with students some aspects of yourself. Now you have a chance to share your own characteristic style and model an openness that may assist students to overcome their natural defensiveness about self-disclosure. Remind students that there are many possible ways of being an effective nurse—difference is not to be feared.

LEARNING TOOL 8.3

Evaluating the Learning Experience

LEARNING FOCUS: Critical Thinking Development

This exercise is designed to help you review both the process and content of your learning through participating in this interactive guide to reflective learning. The process of review and evaluation could be helpful to you and most certainly would be helpful to us.

STUDENT ACTION

Please complete the following evaluation form. Your feedback to us is highly valued.

CONTENT EVALUATION

Using this workbook has enhanced my abilities to do the following:

1. Prepare myself for my clinical practica.

1	2	3	4	5
Disagree				Agree

2. Identify factors that may affect the quality of my learning.

1	2	3	4	5
Disagree				Agree

3. Become more aware of my thought processes.

1	2	3	4	5
Disagree				Agree

4. Become more aware of my feelings.

1	2	3	4	5
Disagree				Agree

5. Interact with my instructor and others involved in my clinical rotation.

1	2	3	4	5
Disagree				Agree

6. Think through complex clinical situations.

1	2	3	4	5
Disagree				Agree

7. Apply my knowledge and awareness of factors affecting client situations.

1	2	3	4	5
Disagree				Agree

8. Provide evidence or validation for my self-assessments.

1	2	3	4	5
Disagree				Agree

9. Discover how to deal more effectively with evaluations and performance feedback.

1	2	3	4	5
Disagree				Agree

Use the following space for your comments about what was helpful and what was not.

PROCESS EVALUATION

My experience with this workbook is as follows:

1. The way the chapters were written encouraged active learning.

1	2	3	4	5
Disagree				Agree

2. The exercises and journal writing supported my learning.

1	2	3	4	5
Disagree				Agree

3. The examples were relevant to my experience.

1	2	3	4	5
Disagree				Agree

4. The ideas in this book were practical and relevant to my situation.

1	2	3	4	5
Disagree				Agree

5. The interactive learning method stimulated my interest in learning more about myself.

1	2	3	4	5
Disagree				Agree

LEARNING TOOL 8.3 continued

Use the following space for your comments about what was helpful and what you suggest we change.

A LITTLE INFORMATION ABOUT YOU

Please circle the appropriate information.

1. Gender: Male   Female

2. Age: Under 20   20—29   30—39   Over 40

3. Learning Status: Student   Instructor

4. Year in Program: _____

5. Type of Nursing Program: Baccalaureate   Diploma   Associate Degree
   Other _____

6. Did you have college or university education prior to entering this nursing program?   Yes   No

NOTES ON USE

Student Use.   Please send these pages (or photocopies) to the publisher:

> *Cathy Esperti, Editor*
> *Delmar Publishers*
> *PO Box 15015*
> *Albany, NY 12212-5015*

Your input will help us further refine the content and process of this book. We look forward to hearing from you. Please feel free to include any memorable moments or turning points for you in your learning as a nursing student that you would like to share. We draw inspiration and strength from your stories and reflections. Thank you for participating in this learning journey with us.

Instructor Use.   You can assist us by collecting completed evaluation forms from your class and forwarding them to us at the address listed in the Student Use section. Your feedback would also be greatly appreciated. You have the day-to-day experience with your students and are in a wonderful position to appreciate the impact this handbook had on them. We would honor your suggestions and criticisms. That is all part of learning. Help us to learn more about what will enhance your role as teacher. Thank you, too, for allowing us to participate in the learning experience with you and your students.

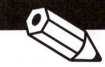

LEARNING TOOL 8.4

Novice and Expert

LEARNING FOCUS: Application Enhancement

A nursing student, in an observer role, reflected on what he had learned from the expert public health nurses he observed.

> *The nurses in the public health clinics were wonderful in their communication skills. They dealt with people who had no English language skills, all sorts of nonverbal skills were used. Special ways of teaching were developed using visual aids to show parents how to care for the baby after the shot.*

Benner (1984) outlined five levels of competence from novice to expert. During this clinical practicum you have gained knowledge, experience, and skill that will help you to advance from novice to other levels of competence. Benner, also, described three criteria that could be used to note advancement in competence: (1) movement from reliance on abstract principles to more concrete experience; (2) increased perception of the factors related to the demand situation; and (3) a movement from primarily an observer to a performer. This exercise will focus on your experiences in each of the five levels of competence.

STUDENT ACTION

For each of the five levels of performance, think about a situation in which you demonstrated that level of competence. Use the three criteria outlined in the previous paragraph to provide a rationale for your choice of that situation. You might also find it helpful to refer back to the Taxonomy of Psychomotor Behavior in Chapter 3 for some descriptions of similar levels of performance.

EXPERT LEVEL OF COMPETENCE

Describe a situation in which you demonstrated the level of proficiency that could be labeled "expert." You can limit the skill or skills which you needed to draw upon, depending upon your clinical experience. For example, you may be an expert at taking blood pressures, but not an expert at interpreting the fluctuations in blood pressure for a specific patient. What criteria did you use to assess your level of competence as expert?

PROFICIENCY LEVEL OF COMPETENCE

Think of a situation in which you demonstrated the level of proficiency that could be labeled "proficient" but not "expert." Again, you may limit the skill or skills you are describing. What more would you need to be able to do to be at an expert level?

COMPETENT LEVEL OF COMPETENCE

This time the situation should demonstrate a "competent" level of performance. How did you differentiate your performance as more than an advanced beginner but less than proficient?

ADVANCED BEGINNERS LEVEL OF COMPETENCE

Describe a situation in which you demonstrated the level of proficiency that could be labeled "advanced beginner." Were there other skills that you used in this situation that were at a more advanced level of competence? What does it feel like to be proficient at some things and not so advanced at others? Do you tend to overlook the more competent skills and just focus on the one that you are learning?

NOVICE LEVEL OF COMPETENCE

Everyone is a novice in new areas of learning. Describe such a situation in which you were a novice. Develop a scale for this skill by outlining what would need to be different for you to be at each of the levels described above.

NOTES ON USE

Student Use.   As you think forward to your next clinical rotation, you can use this way of classifying your skill level to help you assess what learning opportunities may await you. It can also help you develop concrete learning objectives that would indicate advancement in your level of competence in many skills. However, keep in mind always that you are an expert in many ways, in many areas. That is what you will bring to future clinical experiences. Your nursing skills as well as your life skills will all have a place in enriching your nursing care. These reflections might find their way into your practice portfolio for safekeeping.

Instructor Use.   You may be able to provide students with other reference sources that help them assess their progression to "expert." They will need reminding that learning is a lifelong endeavor and that an expert in one area may be a novice in another. Help them to focus on the wider picture of learning and to normalize the wide scope of levels of competence that every nursing student has.

LEARNING TOOL 8.5

The Changing Face of Nursing Today

JOURNAL FOCUS

This is the final journal writing exercise of this handbook. It provides you with an opportunity to reflect upon your understanding of the shift in nursing from an illness and curative orientation to one of care and wellness. This will help you to come full circle within this handbook and move on to new beginnings.

STUDENT ACTION

1. How do you define *wellness*?

2. List several ways in which your definition of wellness could affect the clients you encounter in your clinical experiences.

3. How do you see wellness affecting the "what, when, where, why, and how" of nursing?

4. What difference does seeing the client as a "consumer" of services make to your nursing?

5. Describe the difference between perceiving the person as a "client" or as a "patient" of health-care services.

6. How do you promote wellness in your own life and with those who are close to you?

7. What place do you see for nurses in the legislative reality of health-care reform and restructuring?

LEARNING TOOL 8.5 continued

POSITIVE STATEMENTS ABOUT ME

At the end of each journal entry, you have been drawing out of your reflections and journal writing positive statements you could make about yourself and your learning. You made each statement an "I" statement. We suggest that you gather all of the statements you have made in your journal throughout the past seven chapters and place them together here. This could form a small record of some of your interactive learning.

NOTES ON USE

Student Use.   These reflections will make a great addition to your practice portfolio. Think back to the beginning of this practicum and assess how differently you might have answered the same questions. Write about these changes as a measure of how this practicum has changed your perspective.

Instructor Use.   Have students bring their completed exercises to class. Use their reflections as a springboard for discussion. You might ask them to choose one or two of the questions on which to focus. Remember that they see you as a leader and will be interested in your perspective and how your thinking may have been formed on these issues.

References

Baird, B. (1996). *The internship, practicum, and field placement handbook. A guide for the helping professions.* Upper Saddle River, NJ: Prentice Hall.

Benner, P. (1984). *From novice to expert: Excellence and power in clinical nursing practice.* Menlo Park, CA: Addison-Wesley Publishing.

Burns, De. (1980). *Feeling good: The new mood therapy.* New York: New American Library.

Chubinski, S. (1996). Creative critical-thinking strategies. *Nurse Educator,* 21(6), 23–27.

Dave, R. H. (1970). Psychomotor levels. *In developing and writing behavioral objectives.* Tucson, AZ: Educational Innovators Press.

Kaiser, T. (1997). *Supervisory relationships. Exploring the human element.* Monterey, CA: Brooks Cole.

Montgomery, C. L. (1993). *Healing through communication: The practice of caring* (pp. 106–107). Newbury Park, CA: Sage.

Myers, I. B. (1975). *Manual: The Myers-Briggs Type Indicator.* Palo Alto, CA: Consulting Psychologists Press.

Neufeldt, V. & Guralnik, D. B. (Eds.) (1988). *Webster's new world dictionary of American English* (3rd college ed.). New York: Simon & Schuster Inc.

Perlman, H. (1989). *Looking back to see ahead.* Chicago, IL: University of Chicago Press.

Random House college dictionary (rev. ed.) (1980). New York: Random House.

Rogers, G. & Thomlison, B. (1996, June). *The write stuff: Documenting learning in the practicum.* Paper presented at Conference on Field Education, Ontario, Canada.

Sarasin, L. C. (1998). *Learning style perspectives: Impact in the classroom.* Madison, WI: Attwood Publishing.

Thomlison, B. (1998). Using supervision and consultation. In F. J. Turner (Ed.), *Social work practice: A Canadian perspective.* Scarborough, Ontario, Canada: Nelson.

Thomlison, B., Rogers, G., Collins, D. & Grinnell, R. M. Jr. (1996). *The social work practicum: An access guide* (2nd ed.). Itasca, IL: F.E. Peacock.

Weimer, M. (Ed.) (1997). Learning styles and writing assignments. *The Teaching Professor,* 11(8), 1, 4.

Wright. L. M. & Leahey, M. (1994). *Nurses and families: A guide to family assessment and intervention* (2nd ed.). Philadelphia, PA: F.A. Davis.

International Council of Nurses—
Code for Nurses

The fundamental responsibility of the nurse is four-fold: to promote health, to prevent illness, to restore health, and to alleviate suffering.

The need for nursing is universal. Inherent in nursing is respect for life, dignity, and rights of humans. It is unrestricted by considerations of nationality, race, creed, colour, age, sex, politics, or social status.

Nurses render health services to the individual, the family, and the community and coordinate their services with those of related groups.

Nurses and People

The nurse carries personal responsibility for nursing practice and for maintaining competence by continual learning. The nurse maintains the highest standards of nursing care possible within the reality of a specific situation.

The nurse uses judgment in relation to individual competence when accepting and delegating responsibilities.

The nurse when acting in a professional capacity should at all times maintain standards of personal conduct that reflect credit on the profession.

Nurses and Society

The nurse shares with other citizens the responsibility for initiating and supporting action to meet the health and social needs of the public.

Nurses and Coworkers

The nurse sustains a cooperative relationship with coworkers in nursing and other fields. The nurse takes appropriate action to safeguard the individual whose care is endangered by a coworker or any other person.

Nurses and the Profession

The nurse plays a major role in determining and implementing desirable standards of nursing practice and nursing education.

The nurse is active in developing a core of professional knowledge.

The nurse, acting through the professional organization, participates in establishing and maintaining equitable social and economic working conditions in nursing.

Note: Adapted from the International Council of Nurses. (1973). *ICN Code for Nurses: Ethical concepts applied to nursing*. Geneva: Imprimeries Populaires. Reproduced with permission from the International Council of Nurses, approved by the Council of National Representatives in 1973 and reaffirmed in 1989.

American Nurses Association—
Code for Nurses

1. The nurse provides services with respect for human dignity and the uniqueness of the client unrestricted by considerations of social or economic status, personal attributes, or the nature of health problems.

2. The nurse safeguards the client's right to privacy by judiciously protecting information of a confidential nature.

3. The nurse acts to safeguard the client and the public when health care and safety are affected by the incompetent, unethical, or illegal practice of any person.

4. The nurse assumes responsibility and accountability for individual nursing judgements and actions.

5. The nurse maintains competence in nursing.

6. The nurse exercises informed judgment and uses individual competence and qualifications as criteria in seeking consultation, accepting responsibilities, and delegating nursing activities to others.

7. The nurse participates in activities that contribute to the ongoing development of the profession's body of knowledge.

8. The nurse participates in the profession's effort to implement and improve standards of nursing.

9. The nurse participates in the profession's efforts to establish and maintain conditions of employment conducive to high-quality nursing care.

10. The nurse participates in the profession's effort to protect the public from misinformation and misrepresentation and to maintain the integrity of nursing.

11. The nurse collaborates with members of the health professions and other citizens to promote community and national efforts to meet the health needs of the public.

Note: From the American Nurses Association. (1985). *Code for nurses.* Kansas City, MO: Author. Reprinted with permission from *Code for nurses with Interpretive Statements,* © 1985. American Nurses Publishing, American Nurses Foundation/American Nurses Association, 600 Maryland Avenue, SW, Suite 100W, Washington, DC 20024–2571, p. 1.

C

Canadian Nurses Association—
Code of Ethics for Registered Nurses

Values

Health and well-being   Nurses value health and well-being and assist persons to achieve their optimum level of health in situations of normal health, illness, or in the process of dying.

Choices   Nurses respect and promote the autonomy of clients and help them to express their health needs and values, and to obtain appropriate information and services.

Dignity   Nurses value and advocate the dignity and self-respect of human beings.

Confidentiality   Nurses safeguard the trust of clients that information learned in the context of a professional relationship is shared outside the health care team only with the client's permission or as legally required.

Fairness   Nurses apply and promote principles of equity and fairness to assist clients in receiving unbiased treatment and a share of health services and resources proportionate to their needs.

Accountability   Nurses act in a manner consistent with their professional responsibilities and standards of practice.

Practice environments conducive to safe, competent and ethical care   Nurses advocate practice environments that have the organizational and human support systems, and the resource allocations necessary for safe, competent, and ethical nursing care.

Note: From the Canadian Nurses Association, (1997). *Code of ethics for registered nurses*. Ottawa, Ontario, Canada: Author. Reprinted with permission from the Canadian Nurses Association.

D

Sample Learning Plan

Learning Needs	Intended Learning Outcomes	Strategies, Activities, and Resources	Evidence of Accomplishment

E

Sample Evaluation Form

Nursing Practice Role	Rating	Evidence of Performance
Systematically assesses dimensions of the client experience, using a variety of resources and perspectives.		
Formulates an understanding of client health needs, issues, and desired outcomes, providing rationale and validation.		
Prioritizes health needs and issues in collaboration with client, providing rationale and validation.		
Plans nursing care in collaboration with the client and other members of the health-care team.		
Carries out planned nursing actions based on sound rationale and safe practice.		
Critically reflects on and evaluates the effectiveness and outcomes of nursing care, modifying plans as necessary.		
Uses authentic and responsive relational skills within the caring relationship.		
Implements appropriate and effective health teaching with the client.		
Demonstrates competence with psychomotor skills.		
Develops increasing competence in response to client system issues in relation to individual, family, and community.		

	Rating	Evidence of Performance
Develops leadership skills in client care.		
Collaborates with interdisciplinary colleagues to enhance client care.		
Documents accurate, pertinent information and client observations.		

Professionalism in Nursing	**Rating**	**Evidence of Performance**
Maintains professionalism with clients and colleagues.		
Integrates ethical dimensions into client care.		
Integrates legal dimensions into client care.		
Integrates social dimensions into client care.		
Integrates political dimensions into client care.		

Critical Thinking in Nursing	**Rating**	**Evidence of Performance**
Reflects on clinical practice from multiple perspectives, including nursing knowledge and research.		
Analyzes and synthesizes knowledge from a variety of sources, articulating the impact for practice.		
Critically articulates a nursing framework appropriate to guiding practice in the clinical setting.		

Student Comments:

Preceptor Comments:

Faculty Comments:

Index